Current Clinical Practice

Series Editor
Neil S. Skolnik
Temple University, School of Medicine, Abington Memorial Hospital,
Abington, PA, USA

For further volumes:
http://www.springer.com/series/7633

Neil S. Skolnik
Editor

Electronic Medical Records

A Practical Guide for Primary Care

꽃 Humana Press

Editor
Neil S. Skolnik
Abington Memorial Hospital
Temple University School of Medicine
Abington, PA, USA
nskolnik@comcast.net

ISBN 978-1-60761-605-4   e-ISBN 978-1-60761-606-1
DOI 10.1007/978-1-60761-606-1
Springer New York Dordrecht Heidelberg London

Library of Congress Control Number: 2010936461

Humana Press is part of Springer Science+Business Media (www.springer.com)

Preface

It is not the strongest of the species that survive, nor the most intelligent, but the one most responsive to change.

– Charles Darwin

A virtually awe inspiring idea which becomes the dream of one generation often becomes the reality of the generation to come. At the turn of the twentieth century the United States had 20 million horses and 4000 cars. Gasoline, which was a waste product of the kerosene needed for lamps, was carried in buckets by automobile enthusiasts from whatever source they could find. Over the next decade, a series of watershed events rapidly transformed the car from a novelty to a useful device. In 1903, Horatio Nelson Jackson successfully drove an automobile across the United States, demonstrating the value of the car as transportation. In 1905, Sylvanus F. Bowser perfected the gasoline pump, and the world's first filling station opened later that year. Then in 1908, Ford Motor Company began mass production of the Model T. Coupled with a time of prosperity, the automobile became a lifestyle, available to people of even modest means.

By 1910, there were half a million cars in use in the United States. Unfortunately, breakdowns were still frequent, fuel was still difficult to obtain, and rapid innovation meant that even a 1-year-old car was nearly worthless. The high-wheeled buggy style, directly descendent from the horse-drawn buggy of the previous century, could be driven virtually anywhere. This was necessary, since there were less than 200,000 miles of gravel road and only 1000 miles of paved concrete. It was not for yet another decade, in 1921, that the Federal Highway Act was passed by Congress. This was legislation that coordinated state highways and standardized US road construction practices. Now a century later, we are the proud owners of about 5.7 million miles of paved highway, along with about 125,000 gas stations.

How is this progression of technology, culture, and infrastructure relevant? At any responsible organization new things are regularly introduced. Despite decades of tinkering, electronic medical record (EMR) systems remain a relatively novel technology. The DesRoches data (see Chapter 1) showed that as of 2008, only 4% of ambulatory physicians were using a full EMR, with only an additional 13% using a partial system. There are a dizzying number of models, and they can be taken in almost any direction (even off-road). Features can become quickly obsolete, and the government has just begun settle on national standards for their use. Perhaps most importantly, the entire cultural transformation that attends new technologies is only just emerging for EMRs.

Physicians have many concerns. Will this technology interfere with the humanism and patient interactions that form the heart and soul, if not the science, of medical care? Will the placement of a screen in the room divert the physician's attention from the patient to filling out unnecessary forms and pieces of required data? Will the "narrative" of the illness, the description of the patient's experience, be lost as the representation of disease is narrowed to discrete data fields?

In addition to these humanistic concerns are the more practical concerns surrounding the efficiencies of patient care and the enormous cost of integrating an EMR into a practice. A colleague of ours, Keith Sweigart, focused this issue when, responding to a question about the efficiency of EMRs, he commented, "Remember, the most efficient care is sloppy care." This observation clarified that efficiency, while often discussed and certainly important, cannot be the sine qua non of the electronic medical record. The old practitioner who kept sparse notes about his patients on 3 by 5 inch cards gave humanistic, efficient care; however, the way that practitioner documented his care would never suffice for the complexity of modern medical care, or for the collaborative care that is now necessary in any group practice. As medical knowledge becomes more complex, it will become ever more important to have primary care physicians providing the majority of care for patients, and it will become increasingly necessary to have systems that coordinate a patient's care among all providers. In order to do this, EMRs will need to easily record and transmit medical information in a clear, predictable, and secure fashion between different practitioners.

One of the great potential benefits of EMR systems is population management. Our current system of paper-based individual medical records requires that a physician wait until a patient comes to the office before the opportunity arises to intercede on chronic disease processes. Moreover, the effort to manage risk is often compromised if that patient comes in with another agenda, if they were scheduled for insufficient time, or if the day has become particularly busy. EMRs provide a method whereby we can thoughtfully find those patients who have sub-optimal management and reach out to them proactively.

Through the use of patient portals, EMRs may additionally be able to encourage a more collaborative health system with our patients, who ultimately have the greatest stake in their health care. Patients can access their records and results, dwell over them, and discuss with others how they might address their concerns, in a way not all that different from what we as physicians do during patient care conferences.

Increasingly our method of recording information, in an electronic medical record, will force us to pay more and more attention to the *content* of the information we gather. With this attention to content it is important for us to also keep our focus on the simple fact that the *process* of gathering information and forming relationships with our patients has inherent value. Done correctly, with empathy and attention to detail, this process makes both patient and physician feel more satisfied with the interaction and also affects health outcomes. The relationship that develops between a physician and a patient has a direct therapeutic effect, influences the information obtained, the decisions about what treatments a patient will consider, compliance with medications and lifestyle modification, and keeps the door open so that patients are comfortable returning for follow-up.

The issues surrounding EMRs will not be resolved quickly, or easily. Technology must co-evolve with technique, along with the cultural expectations of patients and physicians. With humanism sustained as the basis of medical care, and with technology enabling the best use of evidence-based medical science, we will improve patient care for individuals as well as the population.

Abington, Pennsylvania   Neil S. Skolnik
Leonardtown, Maryland   Thomas M. Wilkinson

Acknowledgements

Books do not grow quickly. They have a gestation period that is rivaled only by elephants and blue whales. Nor do books develop in a vacuum; they are influenced by their environment and are often facilitated by the discussions, support, and input of others. I feel fortunate to work in an environment filled with colleagues who over the years have also become close friends – Mat Clark, Amy Clouse, Trip Hansen, Pam Fenstemacher, and John Russell – where we help, criticize, compliment, joke, challenge, and ultimately support one other in a way that characterizes and role models for our residents the best aspects of a healthy work environment. This is why, for over 20 years, we continue to have one of the best family medicine residency programs in the region, perhaps in the country, combining core clinical medicine with strong academics and training individuals who go on to become some of the best family doctors in our tri-state area. A program like this, that sees patients from all backgrounds regardless of their ability to pay in an environment of support and respect, can only occur when supported strongly by a parent hospital and the people in charge of that hospital – Jack Kelly, Meg McGoldrick, and now Larry Merlis – individuals committed to doing the right thing for the patients in our community, and Keith Sweigart who led the Abington Memorial Hospital search and launch of an electronic health record.

No plant, no person, and no book grows to its best and fullest without the love and support of family. I save the most important acknowledgements for last, because my last thoughts each day and my first thoughts each morning are about my family – always living I've slowly only noticed the most important things in life – my wife Alison, who I love and with whom I travel together down this wonderful, confusing, cascading river of life; my daughter Ava – who is a delight and whose singing I hear even in my sleep; and my son, Aaron – with whom I have shared the greatest fishing adventures of a lifetime.

Neil S. Skolnik

Contents

Contributors

Kenneth G. Adler, MD, MMM, CPHMS, FHIMSS Independent Health IT Consultant and Practicing Family Physician, Adler Health IT Consulting and Arizona Community Physicians, 5300 East Erickson St. Suite 108, Tucson, AZ 85712, USA, kadler@azacp.com

Catherine M. DesRoches, Dr. PH Department of Medicine (Health Policy), Harvard Medical School and Massachusetts General Hospital, Mongan Institute for Health Policy, Boston, MA, USA, cdesroches@partners.org

Anupam Kashyap, B.E, M.B.A Director of Implementation eClinicalWorks, 140 Broadway, New York, NY 10005, USA, anupam@eclinicalworks.com

Paola D. Miralles, BS Massachusetts General Hospital, Mongan Institute for Health Policy, Boston, MA, USA

Christopher Notte, MD Doylestown Hospital, 1700 Horizon Drive, Chalfont, PA 18914-3950, USA, cmnotte@gmail.com

Neil S. Skolnik, MD Family Medicine Residency Program, Abington Memorial Hospital and Professor of Family and Community Medicine, Temple University School of Medicine, Philadelphia, PA, USA, nskolnik@comcast.net

Thomas M. Wilkinson, MD St. Mary's Hospital, 25500 Point Lookout Rd., Leonardtown, MD 20650, USA, tmwilkinson@pol.net

Chapter 1
Meaningful Use of Health Information Technology: What Does it Mean for Practicing Physicians?

Catherine M. DesRoches and Paola D. Miralles

The first rule of any technology used in a business is that automation applied to an efficient operation will magnify the efficiency. The second is that automation applied to an inefficient operation will magnify the inefficiency.
                                                                                    –Bill Gates

Abstract This chapter addresses the components of American Recovery and Reinvestment Act of 2009 (ARRA), specifically the provisions (collectively labeled HITECH) relevant to physicians practicing in ambulatory settings. Specifically, Chapter 1 highlights the incentives available to physicians through Medicare and Medicaid, as well as proposed requirements for "meaningful use" of EHR systems.

Keywords Meaningful use · Ambulatory physicians · ARRA, HITECH, EHRs · Medicare reimbursements · Medicaid reimbursements · EHR physician incentives

Health information technology (HIT), such as sophisticated electronic health records (EHRs), has the potential to decrease costs, improve health outcomes, coordinate care, and improve public health [1–4]. In recognition of these potential, federal policy makers during the past 5 years have sought to spur the adoption of these systems through executive orders, regulatory reforms, and legislation [5–7]. Since President Bush called for the near-universal adoption of EHRs by 2014, there have been hundreds of pieces of legislation addressing one or more aspects of health information technology, culminating in the February 2009 passage of the American Recovery and Reinvestment Act of 2009 (ARRA) [8]. ARRA contains

C.M. DesRoches (✉)
Department of Medicine (Health Policy), Mongan Institute for Health Policy, Harvard Medical School, Massachusetts General Hospital, 50 Staniford Street, 9th Floor, Boston, MA 02114, USA
e-mail: cdesroches@partners.org

N.S. Skolnik (ed.), *Electronic Medical Records*, Current Clinical Practice,
DOI 10.1007/978-1-60761-606-1_1, © Springer Science+Business Media, LLC 2011

provisions (collectively labeled HITECH) which support the development, adoption, and upgrade of HIT by authorizing new federal investments in HIT capability and use in accordance with the development of federal standards. The act both incentivizes EHR adoption among physicians and hospitals, and establishes a formal policy-making framework to support the development of a nationwide infrastructure that will enable the electronic use and accurate exchange of health information [8].

In this chapter, we review the components of ARRA that are relevant to physicians practicing in ambulatory settings. Specifically, the chapter will highlight the incentives available to physicians through Medicare and Medicaid, as well as proposed requirements for "meaningful use" of EHR systems.

Medicare and Medicaid Payment Incentives

With the goal of markedly increasing the use of HIT broadly and EHRs more generally, ARRA allows for the deployment of both financial incentives and penalties to encourage adoption. In the legislation, the Centers for Medicare and Medicaid Services (CMS) is given the authority to provide monetary incentives to physicians under Medicare and Medicaid to encourage the purchase and use of EHRs. Physicians who do not adopt within the time frame specified by the legislation will be subject to financial penalties (see Table 1.1) in the form of reduced Medicare payments.

Table 1.1 Medicare incentive payments for adoption and meaningful use of certified EHR

Adoption year	First payment year amount and subsequent payment amounts in following years (in thousands of dollars)	Reduction in fee schedule for non-adoption/use
2011	$18, $12, $8, $4, $2	0
2012	$18, $12, $8, $4, $2	0
2013	$15, $12, $8, $4,	0
2014	$12, $8, $4	0
2015	0	−1% of Medicare fee schedule
2016	0	−2% of Medicare fee schedule
2017	0	−3% of Medicare fee schedule

Source: American Medical Association at http://www.ama-assn.org/ama1/pub/upload/mm/399/arra-hit-provisions.pdf; CMS; ARRA Title IV Subtitle B § 4102 (a) (adding new section 1886 (n)(2) to the Social Security Act)

In order to qualify for the incentive payments, physicians must demonstrate "meaningful use" of EHRs, defined by the statute as the following: (1) using a certified EHR technology in a demonstrably meaningful way (e.g., e-prescribing); (2)

using certified EHR technology that allows for the electronic exchange of health information to improve the quality of health care, such as promoting care coordination; and (3) reporting on clinical quality and other measures selected by the secretary of Health and Human Services (HHS) using certified EHR technology [9]. State Medicaid agencies may develop their own definitions of meaningful use; however, these definitions must be approved by the Secretary of HHS. Further, any state definition that differs from the Medicare criteria must address populations in the state with unique needs, such as children, and must be compatible with state or federal administration management systems [10]. Finally, while the secretary of HHS is obligated to implement the Medicare HIT incentives set by ARRA, Medicaid implementation is an optional state undertaking.

Incentives for Physicians under Medicare

The financial incentives available under ARRA are targeted toward physicians practicing in fee-for-service settings, hospitals, and in limited cases, Medicare Advantage (MA) organizations. Any physician may be eligible for the incentives, regardless of their Medicare patient panel. As shown in Table 1.1, beginning in 2011, physicians who can demonstrate "meaningful use" (described below) can receive Medicare payments for up to 5 years, equal to an additional 75% of the physician's allowable Medicare charges for a given year [1, 11]. Practically, this means that physicians who demonstrate meaningful use by 2012 can receive up to $44,000 in incentive payments between the years 2011 and 2015. Physicians adopting by 2013 will receive $39,000, and those who adopt in 2014 will receive $24,000. ARRA also creates additional incentives for physicians practicing in rural health professional shortage areas. They are eligible to receive a 10% increase on the incentive payments described in Table 1.1.

Beginning in 2015, physicians who are not meaningful users of EHRs will be penalized in the form of reduced Medicare fees at the rate of 1% per year. ARRA allows the Secretary of HHS to further reduce Medicare payments by a total of 5% if fewer than 75% of providers are meaningful EHR users by 2018 [12].

Incentives for Physicians under Medicaid

ARRA provides significant financial support through Medicaid for state efforts to bolster EHR adoption. States will be eligible for a 100% federal contribution to enable EHR adoption among several groups of clinicians serving a high volume of Medicaid patients, and in the case of federally qualified health centers (FQHC) and rural clinics, "needy" patients. The following groups of physicians can qualify for incentive payments through Medicaid [13]:

- Clinicians [this includes physicians, dentists, certified nurse midwives, nurse practitioners, and physician assistants in federally qualified health centers (FQHC) or rural health centers (RHC) led by a PA] with a patient panel comprised of at least 30% Medicaid beneficiaries over a continuous 90-day period within a calendar year;
- Clinicians practicing "predominantly" in a rural health clinic or federally qualified health center (FQHC) settings with at least 50% of their total patient volume comprised of "needy" patients. Needy patients include the following: Medicaid enrollees, State Children's Health Insurance Program (SCHIP) beneficiaries, and those receiving uncompensated care or paying on a sliding fee basis; and
- Pediatricians with a patient panel comprised of at least 20% Medicaid beneficiaries over a continuous 90-day period within a calendar year.

Physicians who choose to receive incentives through their state Medicaid program must agree to waive any right to Medicare HIT payments [14].

In recognition that physicians who predominantly serve Medicaid patients may not have the financial wherewithal to invest in new technologies, the Medicaid incentive program makes financing available to these providers for technology implementation and upgrades [15]. Physicians who meet the criteria for serving a high volume of Medicaid patients are eligible for up to 85% of the net average allowable costs for purchasing a certified EHR system, including support and training. There is a maximum of $25,000 for the first year and $10,000 for each subsequent year, over a 6-year period. After the initial start-up payment, all further payments are conditioned on meaningful use of the EHR technology as defined by each individual state.

As shown in Table 1.2, Medicaid incentives begin in 2011 and are provided on a phased down basis. As discussed above, physicians will be eligible for payments to purchase and implement EHRs, as well as incentive payments for meaningful use of these systems. An initial payment to cover the cost of purchasing or upgrading a system, including technology and training, could equal $21,500 (85% of $25,000). Eligible providers may then receive up to $8,500 (85% of $10,000) per year for

Table 1.2 Medicaid incentives for meaningful use (in thousands of dollars)

Adoption year	2011	2012	2013	2014	2015	2016	2017	2018	2019	2020	2021	Total
2011	$21.5	$8.5	$8.5	$8.5	$8.5	$8.5	$0	$0	$0	$0	$0	$63,750
2012		$21.5	$8.5	$8.5	$8.5	$8.5	$8.5	$0	$0	$0	$0	$63,750
2013			$21.5	$8.5	$8.5	$8.5	$8.5	$8.5	$0	$0	$0	$63,750
2014				$21.5	$8.5	$8.5	$8.5	$8.5	$8.5	$0	$0	$63,750
2015					$21.5	$8.5	$8.5	$8.5	$8.5	$8.5	$0	$63,750
2016						$21.5	$8.5	$8.5	$8.5	$8.5	$8.5	$63,750

Source: CMS; ARRA Title IV Subtitle B § 4201(a) (amending Section 1903 of the Social Security Act, 42 U.S.C.A. § 1396b)

5 years of operation and maintenance, as long as they continue to demonstrate meaningful use. Physicians who adopt EHRs after 2016 will not be eligible for incentive payments.

These payments could total up to $63,750 per physician for those with at least 30% Medicaid patient volume. The choice for physicians between the Medicare and the Medicaid incentive program is significant: for early adopters, potential Medicaid incentive payments could be significantly higher than those under the Medicare program [15].

What is Meaningful Use?

As specified in ARRA, "meaningful use of certified EHR technology should result in health care that is patient-centered, evidence-based, prevention-oriented, efficient, and equitable" [16]. But how will this actually be implemented? And how will physicians be required to show that they are using an EHR in a "meaningful" way? In this section, we focus on CMS's approach to meaningful use, with specific objectives that physicians must meet in order to qualify for incentive payments.

Forecasting future plans for updating meaningful use criteria, CMS has taken a phased approach to structuring implementation. Currently in Stage 1, scheduled for 2011 and 2012, physicians must show that they are using an EHR to do each of the following, consistent with other provisions of Medicare and Medicaid law [16]:

1. Electronically capture health information in a coded format,
2. Track key clinical conditions and communicate that information for care coordination purposes,
3. Facilitate disease and medication management, and
4. Report clinical quality measures and public health information.

Meaningful use requirements for Stage 2 have not been finalized.

In order to track progress toward these goals, the HIT Policy Committee (HITPC) established through ARRA has specified five health outcome policy objectives [16]. Within each of these objectives is a set of IT functionalities that must be implemented and measurement goals that must be attained. In response to comments submitted to the interim rule on meaningful use, ONC has divided these elements into two groups. There is a set of 15 core activities that all physicians must achieve in order to qualify for meaningful use incentives. These core objectives are viewed by ONC as the "essential starting point" for the meaningful use of EHRs [16]. There are 10 additional criteria, from which physicians must select 5 to implement during the first 2 years of implementation. The complete list of activities is shown in Table 1.3.

In the following section, we return to ONC's health policy outcome objectives, reviewing each of these activities in turn, examining both the necessary EHR-related activities and the measurement goals.

Table 1.3 Summary of meaningful use objectives and measures for ambulatory physicians

Stage 1 objective	Stage 1 measure
Core set	
Use computerized provider order entry (CPOE)	More than 30% of unique patients with at least one medication in their medication list have at least one medication order entered through CPOE
Implement drug–drug and drug–allergy interaction checks	Functionality enabled for the entire EHR reporting period
Generate and transmit permissible prescriptions electronically	More than 40% of all permissible prescriptions are transmitted electronically using certified EHR technology
Record demographics (sex, race, ethnicity, date of birth, and preferred language)	More than 50% of all unique patients have demographics recoded as structured data
Maintain an up-to-date problem list of current and active diagnoses	More than 80% of all unique patients have at least one entry recorded as structured data
Maintain active medication list	More than 80% of all unique patients have at least one entry or indication recorded as structured data
Maintain active medication allergy list	More than 80% of all unique patients have at least one entry or indication recorded as structured data
Record and chart changes in vital signs (height, weight, blood pressure, body mass index, growth charts for children)	More than 50% of all unique patients age 2 and over
Record smoking status	More than 50% of all unique patients age 13 and over have smoking status recorded as structured data
Implement 1 clinical decision support (CDS) rule relevant to specialty or high clinical priority and the ability to track compliance to that rule	Implement 1 CDS rule
Report ambulatory clinical measures to CMS or to the States	For 2011, provide aggregate numerator and exclusions through attestation and for 2012, electronically submit the measures
Upon request, provide patients with an electronic copy of their health information	More than 50% of requesting patients receive electronic copy within 3 business days
Provide clinical summaries for patients for each office visit	Clinical summaries provided for more than 50% of all office visits within 3 business days
Capability to exchange key clinical information among providers of care and patient authorized entities electronically	Performed at least one test of certified EHR technology's capacity to electronically exchange key clinical information
Protect electronic health information created or maintained by the certified EHR technology through the implementation of appropriate technical capabilities	Conduct/review a security risk analysis, implement security updates as necessary, and correct identified security deficiencies

Table 1.3 (continued)

Menu set	
Implement drug-formulary checks	Functionality enabled and has access to one internal or external formulary for the entire EHR reporting period
Incorporate clinical lab-test results into certified EHR as structured data	More than 40% of all clinical lab tests ordered whose results in a positive/negative or numeric format are incorporated into EHRs as structured data
Generate lists of patients by specific conditions to use of quality improvement, reduction of disparities, and research/outreach	Generate at least one report listing patients with a specific condition
Send reminders to patients per patient preference for preventive or follow-up care	Reminder sent to more than 20% of all unique patients 65 years of age or older or 5 years of age or younger
Provide patients with timely electronic access to their health information	More than 10% of are provided timely electronic access to their health information within 4 business days of its being updated in the EHR
Use EHR-certified technology to identify patient-specific education resources and provide those to the patient as appropriate	More than 10% of patients are provided patient-specific education resources
Perform medication reconciliation between care settings	Perform medication reconciliation for more than 50% of transitions of care
Provide a summary care record for each transition of care and referral to another provider or setting	Provide summary of care record for more than 50% of transitions of care or referrals
Capability to submit electronic data to immunization registries or Immunization Information Systems and actual submission in accordance with applicable law and practice	Perform at least one test of certified EHR technology's capacity to submit electronic data to immunization registries and Immunization Information Systems; follow-up submission if test successful (where registries can accept electronic submissions)
Capability to provide electronic syndromic surveillance data to public health agencies and actual transmission according to applicable law and practice	Perform at least one test of certified EHR technology's capacity to provide electronic syndromic surveillance data to public health agencies and follow-up submission if test successful (where public health agencies can accept electronic data)

Source: HHS and CMS, Medicare and Medicaid Programs; Electronic Health Record Incentive Program; Final Rule at http://edocket.access.gpo.gov/2010/pdf/E9-31217.pdf

Health Outcomes and Policy Priorities: Improving Quality, Safety, Efficiency, and Reducing Health Disparities

Within this objective, physicians must demonstrate that they are using an EHR in such a way so as to improve the quality, safety, and efficiency of the care they deliver.

Further, they need to demonstrate that they are using the technology in a way that will reduce health disparities. In order to do this, physicians must engage in the following activities [16]:

- Provide access to comprehensive patient health data for the patient's health-care team,
- Use evidence-based order sets and computerized physician order entry (CPOE),
- Apply clinical decision support at the point of care, and
- Report information for quality improvement and public reporting.

Table 1.4 lays out the specific objectives and measures related to the care goals listed above. These activities comprise the bulk of the requirements to achieve meaningful use in Stage 2. In total, there are 11 core activities that physicians must engage in within this policy priority and 4 additional activities that they may choose to implement.

Table 1.4 Stage 1 objectives and measures for improving quality, safety, efficiency, and reducing health disparities[a]

Stage 1 objective	Stage 1 measure
Core set	
Use computerized provider order entry (CPOE)	More than 30% of unique patients with at least one medication in their medication list have at least one medication order entered through CPOE
Implement drug–drug and drug–allergy interaction checks	Functionality enabled for the entire EHR reporting period
Generate and transmit permissible prescriptions electronically	More than 40% of all permissible prescriptions are transmitted electronically using certified EHR technology
Record demographics (sex, race, ethnicity, date of birth, and preferred language)	More than 50% of all unique patients have demographics recoded as structured data
Maintain an up-to-date problem list of current and active diagnoses	More than 80% of all unique patients have at least one entry recorded as structured data
Maintain active medication list	More than 80% of all unique patients have at least one entry or indication recorded as structured data
Maintain active medication allergy list	More than 80% of all unique patients have at least one entry or indication recorded as structured data
Record and chart changes in vital signs (height, weight, blood pressure, body mass index, growth charts for children)	More than 50% of all unique patients age 2 and over

Table 1.4 (continued)

Stage 1 objective	Stage 1 measure
Record smoking status	More than 50% of all unique patients age 13 and over have smoking status recorded as structured data
Implement one clinical decision support (CDS) rule relevant to specialty or high clinical priority and the ability to track compliance to that rule	Implement one CDS rule
Report ambulatory clinical measures to CMS or to the States	For 2011, provide aggregate numerator and exclusions through attestation and for 2012, electronically submit the measures
Menu set	
Implement drug-formulary checks	Functionality enabled and has access to one internal or external formulary for the entire EHR reporting period
Incorporate clinical lab-test results into certified EHR as structured data	More than 40% of all clinical lab tests ordered whose results in a positive/negative or numeric format are incorporated into EHRs as structured data
Generate lists of patients by specific conditions to use of quality improvement, reduction of disparities, and research/outreach	Generate at least one report listing patients with a specific condition
Send reminders to patients per patient preference for preventive or follow-up care	Reminder sent to more than 20% of all unique patients 65 years of age or older or 5 years of age or younger

Source: HHS and CMS, Medicare and Medicaid Programs; Electronic Health Record Incentive Program; Final Rule at http://edocket.access.gpo.gov/2010/pdf/E9-31217.pdf
[a] All objectives and measures apply to eligible professionals (EPs)

Health Outcomes and Policy Priorities: Engage Patients and Their Families in Their Health Care

Within this policy priority, physicians must be able to show that they are using an EHR to provide patients and families with timely access to data, knowledge, and the tools necessary to make informed decisions and manage their health. This may include electronic access to test results, records, and discharge summaries. Electronic information may be provided through a number of secure electronic methods including, but not limited to personal health records, patient portals, and external data storage drives, CDs and USB port drives [16]. Physicians may also choose, as one of the five additional activities they must engage in, to use their EHR to identify and provide appropriate patient education materials. Table 1.5 lays out the specific care goals and measurement objectives related to engaging patients and families.

Table 1.5 Stage 1 objectives and measures for engaging patients and families in their health care[a]

Stage 1 objective	Stage 1 measure
Core set	
Upon request, provide patients with an electronic copy of their health information	More than 50% of requesting patients receive electronic copy within 3 business days
Provide clinical summaries for patients for each office visit	Clinical summaries provided for more than 50% of all office visits within 3 business days
Menu set	
Provide patients with timely electronic access to their health information	More than 10% of patients are provided timely electronic access to their health information within 4 business days of its being updated in the EHR
Use EHR-certified technology to identify patient-specific education resources and provide those to the patient as appropriate	More than 10% of patients are provided patient-specific education resources

Source: HHS and CMS, Medicare and Medicaid Programs; Electronic Health Record Incentive Program; Final Rule at http://edocket.access.gpo.gov/2010/pdf/E9-31217.pdf
[a]All objectives and measures apply to eligible professionals (EPs)

Health Outcomes and Policy Priorities: Improving Care Coordination

Under this priority area, physicians must be able to demonstrate that they are able to electronically exchange meaningful clinical information among all "authorized entities" of a patient's care team. The HITPC defines "authorized entities" as any individual or organization to which the patient has granted access to their clinical information. This could include insurance companies, personal health record vendors, or other physicians. The HITPC is cognizant of the fact that in most areas

Table 1.6 Stage 1 objectives and measures for improving care coordination[a]

Stage 1 objective	Stage 1 measure
Core set	
Capability to exchange key clinical information among providers of care and patient authorized entities electronically	Performed at least one test of certified EHR technology's capacity to electronically exchange key clinical information
Menu set	
Perform medication reconciliation between care settings	Perform medication reconciliation for more than 50% of transitions of care
Provide a summary care record for each transition of care and referral to another provider or setting	Provide summary of care record for more than 50% of transitions of care or referrals

Source: HHS and CMS, Medicare and Medicaid Programs; Electronic Health Record Incentive Program; Final Rule at http://edocket.access.gpo.gov/2010/pdf/E9-31217.pdf
[a]All objectives and measures apply to eligible professionals (EPs)

of the country, the infrastructure necessary to support electronic data exchange is not yet available and has excluded the actual exchange of electronic data from the Stage 1 objectives. Eligible providers must simply show that they have the capability to exchange data by performing at least one test of their EHRs' capacity for data exchange. However, in future years, the threshold for these measures will be raised as the capacity for electronic data exchange increases [16]. Table 1.6 presents the specific objectives and measures related to this policy priority area.

Health Outcomes and Policy Priority: Ensuring Adequate Privacy and Security Protections for Personal Health Information

The privacy and the security of electronic health records have long been concerns expressed by patients and policy makers alike. In response to these concerns, and in recognition of the fact that protecting individuals' health information is necessary in order to build public trust in electronic health information systems [17, 18], Congress crafted ARRA to significantly revise health information privacy and security law, particularly the Health Insurance Portability and Accountability Act (HIPAA). The statute broadens HIPAA's reach and strengthens its privacy and security standards, in addition to adding new provisions related to enforcement and entities not covered by HIPAA [19]. The meaningful use criteria contain a provision designed to ensure privacy and security protections for confidential information through "operating policies, procedures, and technologies and in compliance with applicable law" [16]. Specifically, the criteria require that physicians meet the following objective: protect electronic health information created or maintained by the certified EHR technology through the implementation of appropriate technical capabilities (see Table 1.7). There is only one measure associated with this objective in Stage 1. Physicians must conduct or review a security risk analysis and implement security upgrades as necessary [16].

Table 1.7 Stage 1 objectives and measures for ensuring adequate privacy and security protections for personal health information[a]

Stage 1 objective	Stage 1 measure
Core set	
Protect electronic health information created or maintained by the certified EHR technology through the implementation of appropriate technical capabilities	Conduct/review a security risk analysis, implement security updates as necessary, and correct identified security deficiencies

Source: HHS and CMS, Medicare and Medicaid Programs; Electronic Health Record Incentive Program; Final Rule at http://edocket.access.gpo.gov/2010/pdf/E9-31217.pdf
[a]All objectives and measures apply to eligible professionals (EPs)

Health Outcomes and Policy Priorities: Improving Public Health

The final outcome and policy priority is using EHRs to improve public health. Notably, there are no required activities under this policy priority. Physicians may choose, as one of their five additional activities, to demonstrate that their EHR has the capacity to submit electronic structured data to immunization registries and/or provide electronic syndromic surveillance data to public health agencies "according to applicable law and practice" [16]. Table 1.8 presents the specific objectives and measures that are related to this policy priority.

Table 1.8 Stage 1 objectives and measures for improving public health[a]

Stage 1 objective	Stage 1 measure
Menu set	
Capability to submit electronic data to immunization registries or Immunization Information Systems and actual submission in accordance with applicable law and practice	Perform at least one test of certified EHR technology's capacity to submit electronic data to immunization registries and Immunization Information Systems; follow-up submission if test successful (where registries can accept electronic submissions)
Capability to provide electronic syndromic surveillance data to public health agencies and actual transmission according to applicable law and practice	Perform at least one test of certified EHR technology's capacity to provide electronic syndromic surveillance data to public health agencies and follow-up submission if test successful (where public health agencies can accept electronic data)

Source: HHS and CMS, Medicare and Medicaid Programs; Electronic Health Record Incentive Program; Final Rule at http://edocket.access.gpo.gov/2010/pdf/E9-31217.pdf
[a]All objectives and measures apply to eligible professionals (EPs)

Practical Help for Becoming a "Meaningful User"

As this chapter demonstrates, it may seem as though there are many requirements that physicians must meet in order to qualify for incentive payments for meaningful use. In recognition of this, ONCHIT is currently moving forward on two tracks to ease the transition for physicians. First, they have established rigorous certification standards for EHRs. Through these standards, ONCHIT is working to ensure that all certified EHRs can support the achievement of the proposed meaningful use Stage 1 criteria (beginning in 2011) by physicians and hospitals under the Medicare and Medicaid EHR incentive programs [20].

Second, ONCHIT is currently funding the development of Health Information Technology Regional Extension Centers. These centers will offer technical assistance, guidance, and information on best practices to "support and accelerate health care providers' efforts to become meaningful users of Electronic Health Records" [21]. ONCHIT will fund up to 70 of these Centers and each will serve a defined geographic region. The major focus of the Centers' work will be to help select and successfully implement certified EHRs. Recognizing that not all providers will require implementation assistance, the Centers will also be charged with providing the technical support these providers need to achieve "meaningful user" status [21].

Each regional center will work to provide assistance and education to all providers in a region. However, they are directed by ONCHIT to prioritize any direct assistance first to the following groups [21]:

- Public or not-for-profit hospitals or critical-access hospitals;
- Federally qualified health centers;
- Physicians located in rural and other areas that serve uninsured, underinsured, and medically underserved patients (regardless of whether such area is urban or rural); and
- Individual or small group practices that are focused on primary care.

Conclusion

Through ARRA, the federal government has embarked on an ambitious agenda to increase the number of physicians using EHRs to almost universal proportions by 2014. By employing both "carrots and sticks," the legislation aims to move physicians beyond simply implementing a system to using one in a way that will improve the quality, safety, and efficiency of the care they provide, thereby fully realizing the promise of this technology. While the prospect (and the process) may seem daunting, ONCHIT is moving to put structure in place, through certification and technical support, to ease the transition for practicing physicians.

References

1. Blumenthal D. Stimulating the adoption of health information technology. *N Engl J Med.* 2009;360(15):1477–1479.
2. Goldstein MM, Blumenthal D. Building an information technology infrastructure. *J Law Med Ethics.* 2008;36(4):709–715, 609.
3. Lurie N, Fremont A. Building bridges between medical care and public health. *JAMA.* 2009;302(1):84–86.
4. Chaudhry B, Wang J, Wu S, et al. Systematic review: Impact of health information technology on quality, efficiency, and costs of medical care [see comment]. *Ann Intern Med.* 2006;144(10):742–752.
5. Executive Order 13335. *Incentives for the use of health information technology and establishing the position of the national health information technology coordinator.* Washington, DC, April 27, 2004. Available from http://edocket.access.gpo.gov/2004/pdf/04-10024.pdf. Accessed January 04, 2010.

6. Executive Order 13410. *Promoting quality and efficient health care in federal government administered of sponsored health care programs.* Washington, DC, August 22, 2006. Available from: http://edocket.access.gpo.gov/2006/pdf/06-7220.pdf. Accessed January 04, 2010.

7. DesRoches CM, Rosenbaum S. Scanning the health information technology-related policy environment: The promulgation of 'Safe harbor' regulations to incentivize technology adoption. In: Blumenthal D, DesRoches CM, Donelan K, et al., eds. *Health Information Technology in the United States: Where we Stand, 2008.* Princeton: Robert Wood Johnson Foundation; 2008.

8. Rosenbaum S, Cartwright-Smith L, Burke T, et al. Side-by-side chart detailing major health information technology, public health, Medicaid, and COBRA provisions of the American Recovery and Reinvestment Act of 2009. The George Washington University: Hirsh Health Law and Policy Program; March 18, 2009. Available from: http://www.gwumc.edu/sphhs/departments/healthpolicy/dhp_publications/pub_uploads/dhpPublication_C02EEDD2-5056-9D20-3DE547F4F4F83B34.pdf.

9. ARRA Title IV Subtitle A § 4101(a) (adding new section 1848(o)(2)(A) to the Social Security Act), 42 U.S.C.A. § 1395w-4 (West, Westlaw through August 2009).

10. ARRA Title IV Subtitle B § 4201(a)(2) (adding new section 1903(t)(6)(C) to the Social Security Act), 42 U.S.C.A. § 1396b (West, Westlaw through August 2009).

11. ARRA Title IV Subtitle B § 4101 (a) (adding new section 1848 (o)(1)(A)(i) and (o)(1)(B) to the Social Security Act), 42 U.S.C.A. § 1395w-4 (West, Westlaw through August 2009).

12. ARRA Title IV Subtitle B § 4101 (b) (adding new section 1848 (a)(7)(A) to the Social Security Act), 42 U.S.C.A. § 1395w-4 (West, Westlaw through August 2009).

13. American Medical Association (AMA). H.R. 1, the "American Recovery and Reinvestment Act of 2009" explanation of health information technology (HIT) provisions. Available from: http://www.ama-assn.org/ama1/pub/upload/mm/399/arra-hit-provisions.pdf. Accessed January 21, 2010.

14. ARRA Title IV Subtitle B § 4201 (a) (adding new section 1903 (t)(2)(A), (t)(3)(B) and (t)(3)(D) to the Social Security Act), 42 U.S.C.A. § 1395w-4 (West, Westlaw through August 2009).

15. Finnegan B, Ku L, Shin P, Rosenbaum S. Boosting health information technology in Medicaid: The potential effect of the American Recovery and Reinvestment Act. Washington, DC: Geiger Gibson/RCHN Community Health Foundation Research Collaborative; Jul 7, 2009. Available from: http://www.gwumc.edu/sphhs/departments/healthpolicy/dhp_publications/pub_uploads/dhpPublication_506602E1-5056-9D20-3D7DD946F604FDEE.pdf. Accessed January 11, 2009.

16. Department of Health and Human Services (HHS), Centers for Medicare and Medicaid Services (CMS). Medicare and Medicaid programs; electronic health record incentive program. *Final Rule.* Available from: http://edocket.access.gpo.gov/2010/pdf/E9-31217.pdf.

17. Blumenthal D, DesRoches CM, Donelan K, et al. Health information technology in the United States, Where we stand, 2008. Princeton: Robert Wood Johnson Foundation; 2008.

18. McGraw D. "Privacy and health information technology," *in* legal solutions in health reform. Washington, DC: O'Neill Institute for National and Global Health Law, Georgetown Law; 2009.

19. Goldstein MM, Repasch L, Rosenbaum S. Recent federal initiatives in health information technology. In: DesRoches CM, Jha A, eds. *Health Information Technology in the United States: On the Cusp of Change, 2009.* Princeton: Robert Wood Johnson Foundation; 2009.

20. Department of Health and Human Services (HHS), Office of the National Coordinator for Health Information Technology (ONCHIT). http://healthit.hhs.gov/portal/server.pt?open=512&objID=1153&mode=2. Accessed January 21, 2010.

21. Department of Health and Human Services (HHS), Office of the National Coordinator for Health Information Technology (ONCHIT). http://healthit.hhs.gov/portal/server.pt?open=512&objID=1335&mode=2&cached=true. Accessed January 21, 2010.

Chapter 2
A View from the Trenches: Primary Care Physicians on Electronic Health Records

Neil S. Skolnik, Mercy Timko, and Charissa Myers

Do not let what you cannot do interfere with what you can do.
– John Wooden, Basketball coach, UCLA

Abstract It is one thing for pundits in ivory towers to describe the correct approach that practicing physicians should use in selecting and implementing an electronic health record system, for them to describe the essential reasons why it is to the physician's advantage to change over as rapidly as possible to a computer-based system of healthcare. It is another thing to actually make that change. Generals talk about the "cloud of war," by which they mean that even the most carefully developed plans, conceived of in the quiet of the planning room, have to be carried out in a radically different manner than they planned when they face the confusion, disclarity, and realities of the field. This shift from theory to practice is also true of complex systems in medical practice. In the cloud of the office, the physician is often running four patients behind and trying to integrate a patient's psychosocial needs with their medical needs while another patient down the hall is getting an EKG for chest pain. This is occurring simultaneously with trying to understand and integrate the new electronic health record (EHR). It isn't correct to say that knowledge and planning doesn't help; it does and that is why we have written this book. It remains important though to acknowledge that there are different sources available for learning - one is expert opinion and knowledge, the other is experience, the experience of individuals with whom you have something in common and who have decided to implement a system like that which you are considering and to hear their experiences, good and bad, with those systems. The goal of this chapter is to provide readers with candid, first-person accounts of primary care physicians' experiences with a variety of EMR systems from a variety of settings. This should provide a balance of inspiration and consolation regarding a transitional experience that is changing the way medicine is practiced.

N.S. Skolnik (✉)
Family Medicine Residency Program, Abington Memorial Hospital and Professor of Family and Community Medicine, Temple University School of Medicine, Philadelphia, PA, USA
e-mail: nskolnik@comcast.net

N.S. Skolnik (ed.), *Electronic Medical Records*, Current Clinical Practice,
DOI 10.1007/978-1-60761-606-1_2, © Springer Science+Business Media, LLC 2011

Keywords Electronic health records (EHRs) · Electronic medical records · EHR planning · EHR implementation · Aprima software · CHITT certified · e-MD's system · eClinicalWorks

It is one thing for pundits in ivory towers to describe the correct approach that practicing physicians should use in selecting and implementing an electronic health record system, for them to describe the essential reasons why it is to the physician's advantage to change over as rapidly as possible to a computer-based system of healthcare. It is another experience to actually make that change. When looked at from a safe distance, many things fade away and others seem clear. Generals talk about the "cloud of war," by which they mean that even the most carefully developed plans, conceived of in the quiet of the planning room, have to be carried out in a radically different manner than planned amid the confusion, disclarity, exigencies, and realities of the field. This shift from theory to reality is also true of planning for implementation of complex systems in medical practice. In the cloud of the office, the physician is often running four patients behind, and trying to integrate a patient's psychosocial needs with their medical needs while another patient down the hall is getting an EKG for chest pain. This is occurring simultaneously with trying to understand and integrate the new electronic health record (EHR). It isn't correct to say that knowledge and planning doesn't help; it does and that is why we have written this book. It remains important though to acknowledge that there are different sources available for learning – one is expert opinion and knowledge, the other is experience, the experience of individuals with whom you have something in common and who have decided to implement a system like that which you are considering and to hear their experiences, good and bad, with those systems.

The goal of this chapter is to provide readers with candid, first-person accounts of primary care physicians' experiences with a variety of EMR systems from a variety of settings, geographical locations, and backgrounds. Our hope is to provide readers with a balance of inspiration and consolation regarding a transitional experience that is changing the way the medicine is practiced. As the following physicians share their opinions, stories, trials and tribulations, hopes and fears, positive and negative sentiments, we believe one can glen many practical tips and wisdom hard-earned through experience, and perhaps a sense of community.

Interview:
David Dipietro, MD
Buckingham Family Medicine
Buckingham, PA

Dr. David Dipietro is a family medicine physician at Buckingham Family Medicine, practice located right outside of Doylestown, PA. He graduated from Temple University School of Medicine in 1985 and completed his residency at Abington Memorial Hospital. Upon completion of residency, Dr. Dipietro joined as faculty staff at Abington Family Medicine for 2 years prior to joining the Buckingham

Family Medicine practice in 1990. The practice which was once comprised of three physicians has since grown and now houses six physicians, three physician assistants, and has two office sites. The practice, which serves about 20,000 patients, is associated with Doylestown hospital but is owned by three of the six physicians. Each sees about 20–25 patients a day.

My partners and I decided to look into purchasing an EMR system about two and a half years ago. There was a strong push from Doylestown hospital and physicians in the community, who had already transitioned, as well as the governments' reimbursement and an eventual threat of cutting Medicare payments in 2015. It seemed like the right time to do it. We weren't sure what to expect. We brought in a free-state consultant who made recommendations and we reviewed several EMR systems. We then invited those vendors and a few others we had read and heard about to our office to demonstrate how their product worked. They basically walked us through a typical patient encounter. We then narrowed our selection down to two or three vendors and eventually chose one. This took about 6 months. Once we chose our EMR system, the company sent their support team to our office to train us for a few days and they stayed for an additional 2 weeks once we went live. We decided that the EMR system which best suited our needs was Imetica, now called Aprima. The main things we considered when choosing a system were (1) ease in writing notes; (2) others in the community speaking highly of it; (3) good customer support during and after implementation; (4) within our price range; and (5) CHITT certified, which is required for government reimbursement.

We knew that there would be a transition period going from a paper office to a paperless office. The largest challenge with this transition was getting buy-in from the staff. Fortunately, the majority of our staff knew how to type and had some computer knowledge. It certainly changes your practice. Prior to purchasing an EMR, we hoped that it would primarily help to facilitate "stream-lining" certain paths in our office and in the long-run save money by needing less staff to run the office as well as needing less office supplies.

Now, if you were to ask me if my expectations have been met, I'd say certainly not, but I think that's true for most practices. You see, the implementation process takes a few years. That's what people have to be aware of up front. Some people with whom I've talked say that you actually increase your staff as well as your overhead in the first year or two. We found this to be true. In our practice, we've not seen so much elimination of personnel and a shift in their job-title. Where we once had staff pulling charts, they're now responsible for scanning things into the system. I had some idea that this would be the case going into it, but the returns on our investments have been slower than I'd hoped. I'm still waiting on the government reimbursement, and my cost has certainly not decreased as I had hoped.

Initially, having an EMR adds a lot more time to the day and the amount of work I have to do at home. For example, pre-EMR, if I finished seeing patients at 5 pm, I'd be out of the office at 6 pm, but now I'm probably looking at 7–7:30 pm adding about an hour to an hour and a half to my day. I never use to bring work home, now

I bring work home daily adding an average of 4–5 h nightly work that I didn't have before.

So far having an EMR has been a mixed experience. I like that the EMR streamlines a lot of work in our office. For example, in a paper system, when a patient calls the office, the receptionist takes the message, pulls the chart, brings it to the doctor, the doctor writes a message, returns the chart to nurse who calls the patient back with the response, and then the chart is re-filed. With an EMR, the message is sent electronically from the front office to the doctor directly who responds and sends the message back. It cuts down on chart movement around the office. You don't have to worry about not being able to find a chart. Electronic medicine refills are definitely easier. The pharmacy electronically sends a refill to my inbox, I press a button and it goes right out to the pharmacy. As time goes on and charts are retired, there will be less and less pulling of charts and eventually this will save a lot of time and hassle. Another benefit is that notes are typically completed the same day the patient is seen. As a result, turnaround billing is done quicker. Also, if my partner sees a patient and the note is completed by the end of the day it is easily accessible from home. If I'm on call and a patient calls that night or the next day, the note is readily available.

One of the pitfalls of EMR is that it frees up staff time, while more work was now being put back on the physician. It makes it harder on us. I feel like I am doing more work now that used to be done by the nursing staff. For example, refills used to be delegated to the nursing staff, but now refills are done by the physician. This adds more time to your day as a physician. Say you have 90–100 encounters per day (encounters being patients, labs, refills, questions, phone calls) that take only 30 s to a minute a piece to address. Each task does not take long, but since many of these tasks used to be done by staff and are now being done by me as the physician, there is an additional hour and a half added to my day. These little increments of time add up.

With regard to patient interactions, I would say EMR has probably had a negative effect. The EMR takes a getting used to. Its interference during interactions is something you have to be aware of and guard against. You get so caught up with the computer and typing that you have to be conscious and make an earnest effort to maintain appropriate, healthy dialogue with patients. Fortunately, in our office we have laptops so we can face our patients, but I know of many offices that use desktop computers and the physicians have their backs turned to the patient. It is hard to maintain eye contact while typing. Patients seem to be not happy with the EMR, but they too are making the best of it, because they know it's the way to the future.

There are hidden costs to the EMR. During initiation of the EMR, we had to cut back on the amount of patients we saw while we were learning the system and adapting to it. In translation, this resulted in a loss of income. We were forced to scale back for our training period (1–2 weeks) and the implementation period (6 months). We eventually had to get back to where we were before as rapidly as possible. During the implementation stage, we saw two patients per hour which equates to 10–15 patients a day (down from 25). It took about 6 months to get back to full speed. Financially this was too long. This equates to about $100,000 of lost income during that time period. What most people don't realize is that, in addition to the upfront cost and wage loss, there are a lot of hidden costs involved. It's a big investment.

In retrospect, I wouldn't do anything different. I am happy with Aprima and I would choose them again if I had to do it all over again. When I advise others about acquiring an EMR, I emphasize finding an EMR system with good customer support. I would also make sure to go with an EMR system that will likely be around for the long haul. I think one problem today is that there are so many vendors who want to tap into the market. You need a company that is going to be around for a while. It doesn't necessarily need to be a bigger company although bigger is sometimes safer. I think it's important to look at a variety of EMR systems because they are all different and what's good for one practice may not be good for another. In a primary care practice, where time is valuable, you need a system that makes life easier for you and saves your time. This can be as simple as finding a system with the least amount of button clicks, pages to scroll through, and a system which makes writing notes quick and easy.

Life was definitely easier in the paper world. We are now a year and half in and I believe it is going to get better. I see movement in a positive direction. We ran into IT problems (frozen screens, trouble-saving notes, Internet going down) without which things may have gone a little smoother. Most things have been ironed out but IT problems still occur about once in a month. You need to experiment with whatever EMR system you are considering.

Interview:
Lynn Ho, MD
North Kingstown Family Practice
North Kingstown, Rhode Island

Dr. Ho is a family physician in solo practice in North Kingstown, Rhode Island and has been using Amazing Charts since the inception of her family medicine micropractice in 2004. She currently does alpha testing for Amazing Charts. She worked for 14 years in the Community Health Centers of RI as an employed physician prior to starting her own practice. She graduated from New York University School of Medicine in 1986, followed by family practice residency at the University of Rochester in 1989.

Her current solo micropractice consists of outpatient family medicine without obstetrics. She cares for a panel of 750 patients, with 30–50 visits per week, 30–60 minutes allotted per visit, and employs no staff except for herself and a part-time in-house biller. Her practice successfully utilizes multiple technological modalities in addition to Amazing Charts, including open-access scheduling as well as online history-taking prior to in-person consultation. She describes her office as one that is "paperless technology-enabled and patient-enabled." She is on the faculty of the Ideal Medical Practices National Collaborative Project as well as the clinical faculty of Brown University Medical School.

I set about selecting an EMR when I was starting up my own micropractice. It made sense to move to an electronic system at that time. I needed a low-cost system, as my current practice is a low-overhead practice. A no-cost system (such as Practice Fusion or other advertising/data mined "free" EMRs) did not exist at that point. Although there were several open source systems around at that time, I thought that they required too much user effort. In the context of setting up a new micropractice and jumping off the ledge of being employed to being the business owner, in the grand scheme of things, it was just a minor decision to select and implement an EMR.

I expected that the EMR would help with documentation, especially legibility issues and access issues. These expectations have been met and exceeded. Before starting my own practice, I was not aware that documentation was such a costly, timely game that is forced upon us by the healthcare system at large. It took a while and a number of tools to be able to document efficiently. The EMR is not faster than paper, but it is more legible, accessible, and complete. In retrospect, I really cannot think of anything I would have done to better align my expectations with what occurred in reality. I think I was well prepared when I set out to do this on my own.

Implementing an EMR takes time. I would offer this as advice to physicians about to embark on this task. Implementation seems slower than it should and there is a definite and steep learning curve. It generally looks like the bigger the group or organization, the harder and possibly slower it could be. Even for me with a staff of one (myself), a stepwise implementation was in order – unable to go paperless from day 1, I was unable to leverage patient documentation tools until I realized I needed them, for example.

The best aspects of EMR, as previously mentioned, are the legibility, accessibility, and documentation it provides and ensures. The worst aspect of EMR is the utter and total dependence on technology for a working office. If your tech goes down, you are "hosed." This reality has happened in my practice and I've had to move back to paper for a day or so. It makes for long nights on the backend of seeing patients— the times when the technology malfunctions require fortitude. The biggest challenge in transitioning to EMR in my experience was adapting office workflow to EMR. If in a non-solo non-micropractice situation, the most important task likely would be buy-in from each member (physician and non-physician) to the concept of EMR as a whole. Without everyone's investment, it can be cumbersome.

In terms of how the EMR has changed my practice, I would say it's better than it would have been with paper: more efficient and effective, less costly than paper charts which require storage costs and more. I am working currently on registry concepts (outside of my EMR and now within it for quality-monitoring) though I can and do this with a separate non-EMR add-on to the electronic office suite.

I don't really feel that the EMR has affected my interactions with my patients. They are generally wowed by my setup and use of technology. Those who were not impressed have gone away, but they were few in number. Occasionally, I find myself staring at the computer… which I try not to do. This does not happen very often.

If you ask whether I'm happy with EMR, happy is not a word I use around EMR implementation. I could be satisfied – actually, yes, I would say that I am satisfied.

Interview:
Dr. Patrick VanSchoyck
Mingo Valley Medical Group
Tulsa, Oklahoma

Dr. Patrick VanSchoyck is a family medicine physician in Tulsa, Oklahoma. He is also a member of the Oklahoma Medical Reserve Corps and is licensed to aid in FEMA disasters. He has had a direct hand in Hurricane Shelter OKC, opening the Camp Gruber Shelter as well as a Red Cross shelter in Lanai, Hawaii following a dam rupture. He received his Bachelors of Arts and Sciences in Mechanical Engineering at the United States Military Academy, West Point, New York. He served in the US military for 5 years prior to going to the Oklahoma University College of Medicine and did his residency at the Oklahoma Family Medicine Residency Program. Dr. VanSchoyck had firsthand experience with EMR while working for OMNI, an 80 physician primary care system located in Tulsa. It is owned by St. John's hospital, a catholic run 600-bed facility. Five years prior to leaving OMNI, they implemented Practice Partner EMR, but since opening his own practice, Mingo Valley Medical Group, he and his partners have temporarily gone back to a paper chart system which he believes has generated higher revenue than that generated with Practice Partner. He has now been off EMR for two and a half years.

Dr. VanSchoyck thinks although EMR is inevitable, the key question one has to ask oneself is "Who is EMR for, who is it benefiting?"

While at OMNI, we spent about 2 years looking for a system that best suited our needs. We wanted a system that allowed us to print and transmit prescriptions, help with coding, as well as one that had diagnosis-based templates and a reminder system, for example "your patient has CHF, did you start an ACE inhibitor?" The hospital primarily wanted a system that allowed us to send and receive data from their computerized system, including the ER. Prior to purchasing an EMR system, my partner, Dr. Rodney Hollaway wrote his own EMR on a MAC system. In retrospect, it was a much better program than the 1.4 million dollar system we eventually bought. It consisted of three MACs in our office and he made templates that you could manipulate and merge. We didn't have security issues and we didn't have to change anything. It did all functions that are being recommended by today's EMR. The system was eventually removed, probably because it was too functional, not requiring IT enough, and the hospital ran on Windows and I think they wanted all their satellite sites to be on the same system. Although I had some knowledge surrounding the various EMR systems out there from attending annual AAFP conferences where there were various EMR vendors displaying their product, the final decision about what EMR system to purchase was ultimately made by the hospital and we ended up with the least expensive, least functional one. This brings me to an important issue. Although there is a lot of hype about how great EMR is and how well it will benefit the physician, I believe instituting EMR systems are mainly for the benefit of hospitals. The hospitals want to be able to look at your data without your permission. Hospital people are looking through your charts so they can implement pay-per-performance. Hospitals want to own our charts as well as access to patients.

Mingo Valley Medical Group is divided into two offices, one having four physicians and the other having six physicians. The four-physician group has integrated Next Gen EMR. We in the six-physician group are still looking for a system that works for us. Some of the things we are looking for are how many clicks it takes to get the job done. The hospitals don't care about this. If you have more than three clicks your EMR isn't working. Although I am aware of the eventual need for implementing an EMR, one of the things I am looking at is the smart pen. It memorizes everything you write and everything it hears. You then dock the pen to your computer, it gets transcribed to your computer (in your handwriting) and it becomes a permanent part of the chart, a hospital record. There is no question that we can't function without an EMR, but this smart pen is something to consider.

My experience with EMR basically boiled down to a loss of income that I never recovered until I decided to abandon Practice Partner and went back to paper charts. I personally felt that the EMR didn't allow me to work to the top of my degree. A paper system is more reliable. It never goes down. It's easily accessible. With EMR if the electricity goes out or you have a power surge (which happens frequently) the EMR will shut off and you are faced with an office full of patients but no chart to look at. One day, our EMR system went down because someone lost control of their car in a thunderstorm and ran into a tree near our office. Our system was down for a few days. That's why I kept all my charts in my office while at OMNI.

The EMR had a negative effect on patients' relations. All the physicians were too busy typing, often with their backs to the patients, to ever make eye contact with the patients. If they decided to jot down notes and wait until later to complete the EMR, they infringed on their free time and ended up having to take their work home. But of equal importance, you lose out valuable information, like is my patient lying, do they appear frightened or sad, are they favoring an extremity, and so on. You become estranged from your patient. EMR significantly impacted the amount of time each encounter took up. It increased the amount of time it took to have a MA take the patent back to a room, take vitals, and then enter the patients' vitals and chief complaint into the EMR. To bring up the EMR in every room took multiple repeated clicks placing codes and passwords which delayed my contact with the patient. Then by the time I got into the room, the EMR would go into sleep mode and I'd have to re-enter my security information. A chart in a door slot is relatively simple and secure. EMR also affected patient interactions in the sense that it decreased the number of patients seen in a day. Before implementing EMR I'd see on average 24–28 patients a day, after 18 months into Practice Partner, I was still only seeing 18–20 a day. This equates to loss of about $35,000/yr. In addition to income loss, secondary to seeing fewer patients, there were losses due to inadequate coding. In my experience, most EMRs do not rank order the diagnosis for maximum insurance collections or billing. Practice Partner didn't even annotate whether the physician should do a slightly more involved interview in order to get a higher reimbursement. If you have an EMR, my best advice is to insist on a salary. A full-time employee physician in a hospital system is worth about 1.9 million dollars per year. If you are seeing fewer patients with an EMR, which you will be, and if your income is based on production, you won't be able to survive. Our hidden overhead cost was absurd. We paid for frequent IT visits, annual EMR maintenance fees, revenue loss from fewer patients, and the unspoken cost of having to send reports (referrals, labs, imaging, etc.) offsite to get scanned in. This resulted in not only heavy cost but periodic loss of information. We also coded separately, so we had to pay to have our information sent to an offsite billing facility.

With regard to writing and refilling prescriptions, EMR did help to facilitate this process but once again, a process that use to take a mere few seconds (writing out prescriptions), now takes a few minutes. The EMR allowed me to print my prescriptions, but at a remote location which means I still had to leave the room, sign it, then return to the patient's room. I am aware that this is more of a hardware problem rather than an EMR problem but the cost of purchasing the EMR was so great that we could not afford to have printers (and print cartridges) in all the examination rooms. Not to mention, the EMR was never up to date with the list of medications for printing.

On a positive note, Practice Partner made very pretty notes when they are completed. It allowed me to drag FH, SH and PMH from documented in-previous visits and drop them to new encounters. On the down side, once a note was saved on the EMR it could not be removed no matter how wrong it was. Labs would drag onto the wrong patient and we were never able to move them. Not to mention, Practice Partner had fixed formatted diagnosis templates which prevented me from merging two templates into one when a patient had two or more complaints.

I'm an early adopter of technology and actually embraced EMR, but I was very disappointed with the time it took to make the notes, resulting in fewer patients being seen and extra hours of work brought home. All this was known and allowed (by the hospital), despite the HIPPA risk. Theoretically, you can't leave the office without completing charts. So going home and remotely accessing your note is a huge HIPPA risk. A fellow female partner of mine used to see her patients, go home, cook, play with her children before tucking them in for the night, then try and spend time with her husband before staying up until two in the morning completing her charts. She'd come in exhausted nearly every day. Out of the 80 physicians in our network, five left after EMR training period due to discouragement. Two out of eight physicians in my office experienced carpel tunnel syndrome after implementing the EMR. The EMR resulted in highly trained physicians acting as transcriptionists. Ultimately, I had to hire a second MA to be in the room with me transcribing while I interviewed, examined, and discussed the diagnosis and treatment plan with the patient.

Now that I have been on paper charts for 30 months, I am quite pleased with the change. I am still trying to figure out how to integrate technology into the examination room. I am experimenting with pre-printed exam forms that are checked and written by hand using a smart pen and then transcribed on a laptop with character recognition. I use a palm pilot with Epocrates for updated medication information. I am also on a search committee for a new EMR system for our 10-physician group, but so far we have rejected three because they had many of the same problems as we encountered previously. We are still looking for a system that we feel works.

Interview:
Cesar Duque Gomez, MD
San Ysidro Health Center System, Chula Vista Family Clinic
Chula Vista, CA

Dr. Duque Gomez is a family physician and faculty member within the San Ysidro Health Center System, a group of 10 community clinics in central and southern San Diego, CA. He is originally from Columbia and immigrated to US in the 1980s. He attended medical school at the University of Wisconsin, Madison and completed his residency at the Scripps Mercy Hospital in San Diego, CA. His interest in EMRs grew during his time with the San Ysidro System. His special area of interest regarding EMR is primarily end-user training and the broad effects it has either in making an EMR system a success or failure. He is currently playing a major role in his organization's transition to a new EMR system.

Our decision to go with an EMR was mostly economically driven based on grants, in addition to internal and external pressures. The San Ysidro Health Center System was given a grant approximately 8 years ago to select and implement an EMR. There was no physician participation in this endeavor. Companion EMR was selected by the administration, the choice was purely cost-driven, and to be used by 110 physicians within the system. At first it was selected and implemented in only one clinic, which also happened to be the site of our residency program. The 8 years that have passed with the current EMR have been filled with frustration and struggle for the physicians working within our current system. I and one of my colleagues have achieved superuser status in effort to help others learn the system from within, but the struggle has continued. Because of this negative experience, a committee was formed specifically to handle new EMR selection and implementation and we sought the help of the Council of Community Clinics. The Council has reviewed many EMR products and has a good knowledge base. The San Ysidro Health Center System is currently in the process of choosing between Nexgen and eClinicalWorks. This will be funded by grants from the federal stimulus package.

The selection process this time around has been very interesting and entirely different with physician or "end-user" input playing a major role. Physicians comprise 40–50% of the committee and have strong leverage, in addition to administrators and medical records personnel who also have valuable input. As mentioned before, both external and internal forces play a role in this process. As a public state clinic system, there are extensive reporting requirements, mainly of demographic data, that the selected EMR would need to meet for this system. Nexgen has great reporting and data mining capabilities, but eClinicalWorks is more user-friendly for physicians. We are trying to choose between the two systems. We do not want to sacrifice physician–patient interaction and healthcare delivery for better demographic reporting.

We have been doing site visits, observing different EMRs in action, speaking with physicians using them, and test-driving them. This experience has given us much hope for implementation of our next EMR, but by no means do I expect a perfect experience. In general, I feel that the common expectations for EMRs including increased efficacy, revenue, and reporting as well as decreased loss of charts and decreased paperwork are not being fulfilled. Efficiency is not better, revenue is about the same or less, and paperwork may be reduced, but certainly still exists. Regardless of the EMR being used, myself and many physicians can still work faster with paper charts; "end-user speed" is the final denominator. At best with an EMR, I may see 11 patients per half day session; with paper charts I could see 24 patients in the same amount of time. Voice recognition does not help in my experience. There is still paperwork. Revenue has not increased: while coding and collection may be more precise, the decline in the number of patients seen more than takes away any ground gained. Currently, reporting is not improved with San Ysidro's current EMR, as the EMR and practice management programs cannot communicate. And while paper charts may no longer be lost, when the EMR system goes down between 1 and 3 h on average per 40 h work-week, the catch-up and backlog of patients and charting is tremendous – it was as much as 5 h prior to superusers being trained to help. Such crashes led to irate physicians within the system calling the system supervisors and contributing to an overall poor morale.

Exercising more forethought and involving physicians heavily in the selection and implementation process as well as investing more resources in user training would be key to having the next implementation successful. Careful selection followed by implementation is the most critical step and it must be most carefully planned. User training is also a key; if one can't use the system effectively, then the system is not very useful. Physicians as the key end-users should be very involved from the very beginning through to the more complex tasks and challenges such as the creation of templates and automated medication lists that they will be using constantly. An implementation not planned carefully can result in templates and patterns set that may not be user-friendly and may even be detrimental.

My advice to those departing on this journey of selecting EMR is to be vigilant and deliberate. Plan carefully, investigate, go and watch EMRs being used in real life, and talk to those working with them everyday. Be thoughtful about every aspect of implementation. San Ysidro has plans for phasing in physicians gradually; at my clinic we have three attending physicians and a large residency program. We anticipate it being a challenge for those who are not computer-savvy. The extra time and resources invested in training users thoroughly, resulting in confident users with a solid foundation, will go as a significant way to a smooth transition for us.

The best aspects of having an EMR include ready access, the possibility of remote access, and e-prescribing which is a tremendous useful tool. Easy access to lab results and notification of urgent results are extremely valuable as well. On the contrary, lack of reliability, which is system-specific, tops my list of the worst aspects of using an EMR. When the system is down, everything is down. As mentioned before, other challenges include the decrease in productivity due to end-user speed, charting taking longer time, and resultant drop in number of patients seen. I think it can also significantly cut interaction with patients; with more physicians focusing on the computer screen, patients will often stop talking, and the overall nature of the encounter can take on a far less personal tone. The interaction time is cut often due to the increased need for time for charting. An additional concern for us as a residency training site includes impact on the residents' graduate medical education/training; they often get frustrated while trying to use the system, resulting in less time and energy for learning medicine, less interaction with their patients, and an overall sense of being rushed and distracted.

The bottom line is that the EMR we currently have and are about to abandon has changed our practice in negative ways: it is archaic; we had no role in selecting it; it has resulted in decreased productivity, decreased efficiency, and increased physician frustration. Yet, out of this negative experience, we have reaped much wisdom and we are hopeful for the next one to be better; not perfect, but better – with a smarter, smoother implementation process and a chance at working through the system, working out glitches, and reaching a point of steady equilibrium and productivity without sacrificing physician–patient interaction and quality of healthcare delivery which must remain as our utmost ideal and most important goals.

Interview:
Mark Cohen, MD
Lifetime Health Medical Group, Perinton Health Center
Pittsford, NY

Dr. Cohen has been practicing internal medicine and pediatrics since 1989. He is the Chief of Internal Medicine, Chief of Healthcare Informatics, and Chair of Clinical Excellence in the Lifetime Health Medical Group in upstate New York. He is a 1985 graduate of Hahnemann University School of Medicine and completed residencies in internal medicine and pediatrics at Albany Medical Center Hospital in 1989. The by-line to his e-mails is "Failure is not an option." With this sentiment he has championed EMR and guided the implementation of a system for 700 employees, 12-location primary care medical organization, which serves more than 100,000 patients.

In 2003, my organization, Lifetime Health Medical Group, started planning for the selection and implementation of an EMR. First, I was given the task of selecting one, so I started searching the web and reviewing demo CDs. Soon the organization had decided to merge several large healthcare groups in three upstate NY cities, and simply adopted the system, Nexgen, already being used by one of those groups in Syracuse. What I discovered was that the system being used was not actually being used as an EMR, but simply as a practice management system. The information technology department had implemented it, modified it to work in conjunction with paper charts, and bypassed the EMR functionality all together. Within a year, I attended a user group meeting for Nexgen to learn about the system in detail from those already using it. Nearly 4 years later in February 2007, after multiple presentations at Lifetime, demonstration, and getting approval for the investment of 2 million dollars, the system as an EMR was implemented – a process which then took 18 months.

Implementation necessitated developing two entirely different plans for offices in the cities of Rochester with four medical centers and five offices which were entirely paper-based, and in Buffalo where four offices were already using a text/DOS-like EMR with dictation. I worked very closely with the administration in guiding the implementation process. A steering committee was formed. The decision to go with a wireless system was one of the first and most important decisions made – for mobility and ease within sites, not necessitating logging in and out constantly to preserve privacy and security, and to prevent the circumstance of physicians looking at walls rather than their patients. The Buffalo site, already using an archaic system with hardware, replaced one element at a time with new applications and modules being unveiled as time progressed. Rochester, starting from paper charts, was transitioned site by site. Entire medical records were scanned for approximately 100% of patients at the Rochester site and 80% of patients at the Buffalo site. All paper records were destroyed.

Laptops with touch screen options were introduced; template clicking versus free-typing is optional, and all physicians were trained on Dragon voice recognition for the option of dictation. All can type, click, or dictate, although free-typed information will not be available for data mining. The lab interface is enormously helpful. The paper trail that used to take up to 2 weeks from start to finish can now take less than 8 h, from physician review of a result to the patient being informed. In transitioning, at one of our health centers, we now need only one person instead of three to manage incoming paper documents, with things growing even faster now that most lab results are coming electronically.

Detailed workflow studies were conducted over considerable time for front-desk staff, nursing, PA's, and physicians. Training modules were issued to every staff member. Training is by far the single most significant factor in success of transition and implementation of an EMR. Accommodations must be made for individuals' differences in learning, in prior experience with technology, and speed in acquisition. Every person received 10 h of traditional classroom training and a manual; this was followed by having support staff shadow the staff member in vivo while working, with support staff in-house for 2 weeks. All schedules were cut by 50%, from four patients per hour to two patients per hour, with no annual physicals included. Over time, information sessions were held for questions/issues and idea sharing. Superusers or "physician champions" were trained. I still work in this role and feel that the essential time for physicians and healthcare workers to learn and the time when they will truly remember how to use the EMR for various tasks is when they are at the point of care, needing to get something done. The Rochester site saw an attrition of two physicians who left because of the EMR implementation.

We expected the EMR to effectively remind and prompt healthcare providers regarding health maintenance issues, patient monitoring, etc. It did not! It is very good at recording, having all information at your fingertips at all times with nothing "getting lost," as can and does happen in the paper chart world. Incorrect "filing" is extremely rare with EMR as there is a double-check of scanning and electronic records that makes the EMR more complete and exact; there are no storage issues and no "chart mistakenly filed within another chart." The beauty of EMR is that information is available to everyone who wants or needs it at all times. Nurse, physician and front-desk staff can all be accessing the same chart at the same time for various purposes. Communication can also occur via the EMR leaving no need to go and find physically a nurse or desk staff member to perform a task. Other benefits include the ability to finish charting from home or other locations outside the worksite; total access anywhere at anytime. The system has become a data mining goldmine with the ability to run queries and perform quality tracking very easily. We use CINA, a data aggregator which mines data, scouring the patients' records and provides a one page summary of the patient's action items.

As far as advice for physicians about to embark on the task of selecting and implementing an EMR, I would say the following: Go to user group meetings. Talk to people. Visit sites and watch the system in action. It is worth the investment. There are drawbacks that one must expect. When the system goes down, e.g., the router has a bug, electricity is out (e.g., squirrel ate through wires which really happened to us!), or interference from nearby wireless networks, the system is down and things grind, at times, to a halt. There is maintenance that must take place. Upgrading templates can require more than 1,000 h of testing before committing to them.

EMR has certainly changed our practice. It has increased revenue and increased number of patients seen (30 per day). It provides us with electronic reminders and prompts that improve safety. Refills via Surescripts are done with ease and with good safety assurance with suggestions, reminders, and prevention of duplication. The data aggregator has contributed tremendously in improving vaccination administration.

I cannot say it has not changed interactions with patients – it's another entity in the room. I approach it in this way: I show the computer to patients and don't use it as a shield. I use it to show them their information and as a way to involve them in their healthcare. Am I happy we now have EMR? Well, I would never go back. Patients like it, information is available easily, it is cutting-edge, and can show patients things about their health graphically in a way that just was not possible with paper charts. When a good system is implemented wisely and used actively with an eye toward improvement at all times, it improves our ability to do our jobs, to improve patients' health and the care they receive, at the bottom-line.

Interview:
Robert Clark, MD
Clark Family Medicine
Newland, NC

Dr. Robert Clark has been practicing family medicine with obstetrics since 2000. He earned his MD from University of Texas Health Science Center at San Antonio in 1997. He established Clark Family and Obstetric Care in Linville, NC after completing residency at Moses Cone Family Medicine Residency Program, where he served as Chief Resident in his final year. In 2006, he moved his practice, now known as Clark Family Medicine, to Newland, NC.

Dr. Clark has an extensive background in information technology preceding his training and career in medicine, which provided him with specific skills and knowledge to begin exploring the world of EMR prior to finishing his residency. He holds a BS in Computer Science earned from Appalachian State University in Boone, NC in 1986 and worked for Texas Instruments in Dallas, TX as a programmer/systems analyst from 1986 to 1991 as well as in Voice Control Systems in Addison, TX as software engineer from 1991 to 1992. Dr. Clark has had articles published in AMA News and the Family Practice Journal regarding the basic EMR he programmed for Moses Cone Family Medicine Residency.

Medicine is my second career. I received my BS in Computer Science from Appalachian State University and began my computer programming/systems analyst career at Texas Instruments in Dallas, TX. With a background in computers, I knew I wanted to have an EMR to make my office flow efficiently. After researching the vendors available in the late 1990s, I opted for e-MDs as the process of software development was the way I would have created a software company to produce an EMR. I used e-MDs as a PGY-3 to record all my outpatient encounters, so I would be ready when I started my own rural practice.

My wife received her MBA and worked in the information technology industry as well. She was a natural to be our business manager. We opted to scan the most current notes (usually about 1 year) along with the lab and test results into our EMR from old paper charts as new patients came to our practice. This made implementation a bit more challenging, but otherwise it went fairly smoothly. We had opened a brand new office and did not inherit paper charts – we started our practice from day one with an EMR. Of course, I created all my notes with e-MDs and added entries as new patients arrived. Labs and tests that I ordered still had to be scanned when we opened our family medicine practice in 2000. Our support staff took to the EMR well. All had experience in other offices with paper charts and quickly came to realize the benefits of an EMR. We ran our office of 25–30 patients daily with a total staff of four, including myself and my wife for about 2 years. I do not believe we could have done this without an EMR.

We started our search for an EMR when I was a PGY-2. After researching online, we determined it was best to see demos and meet the developmental and support staff directly. The largest gathering in 1998 was TEPR in Washington, DC. My wife and I attended and looked at several vendors. e-MDs struck both of us as the most intuitive and had great staff. They offered a free version for residents, which I used during my PGY-3 outpatient rotations. That solidified our choice.

Not being one to enjoy sales pitches, we already had the basic knowledge to select an EMR and felt astute at ignoring "vaporware" promises. That is, we knew we wanted to choose a vendor who had a good business development plans and excellent technical/support staff with a system that worked from day one. Our selection of e-MDs was also based on it providing a fully integrated system, which included billing, scheduling, and charting. Our software experiences had revealed many of the problems with using software components from different vendors. You almost always got the response, "It must be the other guy's software" when problems arose. That can be extremely frustrating as the time demands of medicine do not allow you to tease the real answer out. Our experience was mostly self-generated and very satisfactory.

My expectations for EMR have their roots in my residency which was excellent but had paper charts like almost every other practice in the late 1990s. The frustration of lost charts, flipping through to find results, dictating then waiting several days for a paper copy, and the inconvenience of showing patients their information (e.g., no way to do flow sheets on lab data points easily) was something I wanted to avoid in a new practice. I knew my EMR would avoid almost all of that. I could bring up a patient's chart in the exam room, review trends in labs and test results, print out patient education handouts for specific problems, limit drug interactions through automated checking, and see charts on-call from home. I could limit the number of staff members and overhead by doing my own coding, avoiding space for paper charts, and streamlining patient flow along with their information.

The EMR largely met my expectations. Use of templates took some time to determine best use. Nothing is faster than dictating. However, there are no data points that can be used later for recurring visits. Thus, the initial effort of putting in the template information paid off on return visits. The difficulty is carving out the time needed to do this in a busy primary care office initially. It meant many late nights and missed time from family.

Not being so busy is about the only way I can see the transition to EMR being easier. However, the bills have to be paid and you want to be growing your practice. I believe my expectations were pretty much in line with the reality. Modifying templates to meet my own workflow ended up helping overall. However, I am not sure I would have known that without going through the day-to-day practice activities using the EMR. Maybe having contact with an experienced provider who had implemented the EMR could have been beneficial. However, in 2000 there were not many providers using my EMR.

In terms of advice for other physicians entering the EMR world, working with the software ahead of time is somehow tremendously beneficial. Working with software on a small subset of patients was very helpful as I used it on a much more limited basis as a PGY-3. Develop a team of front and back-office staff who understands the importance of EMRs. You will need frequent meetings to review problems as well as solutions.

The convenience of pulling up a patient's full chart from any location is one of the best aspects of an EMR. Whether I am in the office or at home responding to a page, I can find out the patient's history, what has been done through our office (including other provider's office notes and labs/tests), current medications/allergies, and can document the encounter immediately. I can send prescriptions from anywhere and have eliminated all prescription pads. Additionally, the billing cycle is much cleaner and quicker as the invoice is built prior to patient checkout and our EMR "scrubs" our claims before being sent to the insurance company. This requires only part-time billing staff overhead.

Our labs are electronically placed in flow sheets for my review as well as sharing with the patient without manual intervention. I believe this has motivated patients with hard data to improve in some of their chronic conditions. Finally, patient registries are easy to develop from our database. When medication recalls occur, we run a report to determine who needs to be contacted. We can determine who is at goal for certain conditions on a practice-wide basis. When new medication interactions are found (e.g., Plavix and PPIs), it is easy to find out whom we need to contact to change medications.

One of our greatest challenges having an EMR includes not having electronic connections to specialists and hospitals and the time it takes to print our notes and fax. In addition, we have to redirect electronic faxes to the correct patient in our system when the patient is evaluated by a specialist or discharged from the hospital. On review, I have to update our lab flow sheets and health summary to ensure we do proper follow-up. An electronic data exchange, as is done in many industries, would help my care of patients and save us time and money.

Having EMR has changed our practice: it is much more efficient with higher quality of care and reimbursement than the paper chart environment that I experienced mostly during my residency. In terms of effect on physician–patient interaction, I was initially concerned that this would present some challenges and be burdensome. However, I found that the patients were quite impressed with the use of an EMR. They reported with more confidence in our practice. Sharing data from the EMR, including labs, tests, and patient education handouts, has increased our quality and helped to motivate patients to change for the good of their health. I have found no significant negatives.

If you ask am I happy with EMR? Absolutely! I cannot imagine practicing without our EMR.

Interview:
Dr. Jim King
Family Medicine, Primecare Medical Center
Henderson, Selmer, and Adamsville, TN

Dr. Jim King is a family medicine physician in Tennessee. He received his medical degree from the University of Tennessee College of Medicine in Memphis and completed his residency training in family medicine at the UT Family Medicine residency program in Jackson. In 1985, he completed his residency and moved to Selmer with his wife and three kids and joined his father's practice. That practice later became known as the Primecare Medical Center. Dr. King still works at Primecare and the staff now comprised seven family medicine physicians, one general internist, and three nurse practitioners. They have offices in Henderson, Selmer, and Adamsville, TN. The practice has about 20,000 active charts. In the past 25 years of practicing medicine, Dr. King has held many leadership roles including President of West Tennessee Consolidated Medical Assembly, Tennessee Medical Association (TMA) and Tennessee Academy of Family Physicians (TAFP). Dr. King also has the distinction of being only the second family medicine physician from Tennessee to be the President of the American Academy of Family Physicians (AAFP).

We decided for transition to EMR after hearing all the information presented to us by AAFP and others in our community indicating that technology is changing and we have to move in that direction. One of our partners was interested in computers so that helped us as well. The entire process of selecting and incorporating EMR took about 6 months. We reviewed several systems to begin with and eliminated them based on two criteria: (1) we wanted a company that we were sure would be around for 10 years and (2) the accounting system and EMR had to be from the same system. (We didn't want one group telling us it was the other's problem. Like one group responsible for software and the other hardware.) The experience of selecting an EMR was not very painful but definitely complicated. There were so many variables and so many companies out there that you always felt like you were comparing apples to oranges.

I didn't have a ton of expectations going into it but I knew for sure that it would cost me more money than the system we already had in place and it would slow me down. On the positive end, I believed that it would provide me with better data. I anticipated that it would allow me to document better what I do, resulting in higher level of coding and better reimbursements. I was also hoping that it would give me reminders about things such as immunizations, screening tests, etc. In retrospect, EMR has met many of my expectations but not all, our expenses did go up and our productivity did go down. It took longer than expected to reach an acceptable productivity level, and even still I don't believe we will ever see as many patients in a day again. Prior to EMR, I would see an average of 35–40 patients a day, now I see 30–35. In my opinion, EMR will never make you more money but somewhere between 9 and 18 months you should at least be back to where you were. Of benefit, we are able to code higher because of system documentation.

It's funny how expectations and reality don't always line up. I really thought that I would just turn on the EMR and most of the features I wanted would appear and I would only need to use the ones available to me, but that was not the case. The vendors come out and sold us on their product but they really didn't take the time to determine what we needed. The most frustrating thing was that it seemed like everything we wanted, including but not limited to, e-prescribing, webpage interactions, disease registries, protocols, and flow sheets all had to be added separately and usually for an additional cost.

I am not sure if any of these misalignments of expectations and results could have been avoided, but I would have definitely talked with trainers and service people associated with each product rather than salesmen who may not have always had our best interests in mind.

As I expressed earlier, implementing a new system of any kind can be challenging for a practice, but the challenges can be minimized by adding something new on a regular basis and having a plan on how you're going to implement in place prior to starting. I really don't think we could have done it better. Everyone was up and running in less than 2 weeks. We were moving slow but we were moving forward nonetheless. The largest challenge during this transition was getting all of my partners and staff to agree that EMR is inevitable and that we must all be on board in order for it to work. Once getting past the inertia everything moved better. My advice for physicians who are thinking about purchasing an EMR is to stop hesitating and take the next step, no matter what it may be for you.

In my experience thus far, the best aspects of now having an EMR is that my patients are getting better care. We are following preventive services better, their chronic conditions are managed better, and I can read my partners notes. EMR does have an effect on patient interactions both positive and negative. Because I spent more time looking down and typing, I had to work extremely hard to make sure it didn't appear that I was just a data entry person and not their doctor. But my patients seem to be very receptive and appreciative of EMR. They are impressed when I can look up the latest treatments right there in the room.

All in all I am very much pleased with our decision to implement EMR and I will never go back to paper charts.

Interview:
Keith Sweigard, MD
Internal Medicine Associates of Abington Abington Memorial Hospital
Abington, PA

Dr. Sweigard is the Chief, Division of Internal Medicine and Director of the AMH Physician Network at Abington Memorial Hospital. He has special expertise and research interests in medical informatics and has served as a liaison between the medical staff and the IT services at Abington since the early 1990s.

I have been involved with bringing information technology to Abington since the early 1990s, working as a liaison to the IT department while practicing internal medicine and attempting to bridge the worlds of medicine and IT and maintain those bridges through many transitions over the years.

The early experiences with this process were difficult. We had two failed attempts at trying for transition of our entire physician network to EMR. The first attempt was to use the EMR provided by the same vendor as our patient management system. There was significant performance issues, specifically challenging was the lack of a template design utility. The company had no experience with this. We moved to a web-based application which presented significant data integrity issues, specifically dates not carrying over. We attempted to select a more established EMR, one with a longer history and good track record and in this process physician involvement was increased many-fold as the importance of end-user input was clearly manifest by this point.

We chose the fastest growing vendor who already had systems established in many large settings. We conducted site visits, including a site in the New

York city, to see the system in action, to assess the workflow, and selected eClinicalWorks ultimately. Other factors that led to this selection included the availability and possibility of enhancements for the system. With an eye toward the future and pay-for-performance coming up, we wanted to be secure in improving our population management, our ability to trend, mine data, and use it for the betterment of our care of patients while meeting these new expectations of measures of service. eClinicalWorks as a vendor demonstrated its willingness to innovate for end users and this contributed significantly to our selection of the system.

In practical terms, workflow is one of the most critical parameters in the office setting and selection of an EMR and how it will facilitate or hinder workflow must be carefully considered. What adjustments need to be made once an EMR is implemented must be anticipated so that workflow will continue as smoothly and efficiently as possible. Staff comfort with the system is critical; it leads to better interaction with the patient and all things follow from that. We have had success with data entry, data review, and population management with this system. We still have some performance issues which can be difficult to tolerate in a high-paced office, but having a plan in place for addressing such issues and events is key to fruitful resolution of such events.

Increased dependence on a complex information management system, any technical system really, leads to a very real increased risk of single-point failure. This must be acknowledged, and safety measures and plans must be put in place and reviewed regularly in case of such events. Complex systems will fail. It is not a matter of if, but when. For these reasons, it is essential that all those who are involved keep engaged in day-to-day performance issues and that there may be redundancies built in the system. One must always keep in mind the possibility of larger events such as servers being down, in addition to day-to-day events.

Many clinicians are concerned about what implementation of technology will do to the human interaction that is at the core of the practice of medicine for the physician and the receipt of medical care by the patient. While protocol use is important in patient care and will help us keep better track of parameters measuring quality of care through patient tracking and assessment, some argue this will threaten the human aspect of this interaction. I argue that use of information systems could in fact, paradoxically, improve humanism in medicine. I am very excited, for example, about the future of "patient portals" which will facilitate a more "patient-centric" healthcare system. It will increase patient's understanding and ability to self-manage by involving patients in their own care as partners with us. Being able to review clear med lists, track blood pressure reading, and view such measures on clearly plotted accurate graphs will likely open patients' eyes and involve them in a new way through knowledge and ultimately understanding.

I find that patients are expecting more and more of the use of technology in their care. As a clinician, I try to engage patients with the computer in the room. I show it to them, view it with them side-by-side, looking at med lists, for example. It is not a barrier in my practice. I hope it will make us all better physicians through care reminders and extra support measures. We all need reminders as the world of medicine and sheer volume of information grows even larger, more detailed, and complex.

Another significant issue very close to the patient is that of privacy. Our system currently has an open architecture. Safety and privacy can be at significant odds and can present significant challenges. Do we keep the open architecture and have an audit trail of who has seen the record, with the ability to discover and cite any individual who should not access the record under HIPAA as the policing factor, while allowing those with a need to know for patient care and safety the access they need? We can go too far in either extreme – protecting privacy to the point where it threatens appropriate care by being so cumbersome and presenting points of significant potential danger to the patient. Yet, we must preserve privacy as a fundamental principle of medical ethics. Patients must feel safe in the context of their receipt of healthcare and this sense of safety includes feeling that their privacy is preserved.

My advice for those in the process of considering or selecting an EMR is to look at large vendors with a great install base. The system needs to do all core things well: from e-prescribing to ease of documentation. Consider the big debate regarding template usage versus free texting. Templates work well for diseases, but not for the illness the patient experiences. It is therefore essential to have both capabilities. Structured data including past medical history, medications, and allergies work well. But one must always have the ability to quote a patient regarding his or her own illness experience. You should be able to access results with reasonable ease. This should offset your data entry burden.

EMR is the clear path to the future for all of us in medicine. To the pay-for-performance and quality of care measures, we all will be held to for the betterment of our patients' well-being. Look for a system that provides population management options with a usable tool, easy messaging ability and plans, at least, for patient portals in place. If you don't have good typing skills, acquire them STAT. I would strongly advise anyone not to rely on voice recognition systems; they are far from perfects and because of this they present some significant challenges, words not intended, miscommunications in addition to very clear privacy issues when a clinician is openly verbalizing patient encounters.

In transition, you should make plans for chart storage. I recommend starting to scan paper charts on the first day of EMR implementation. The office schedule must be cut; otherwise the risk of errors is significant. Teamwork is an absolute must. All members of the office staff and clinical care staff must work as a team with the in-house technological support staff. A well-thought out plans must be in place for the human aspect of going through this transition, i.e., for handling and limiting the stress that will incur, for improving communication. Office huddles, frequent debriefing sessions are essential for addressing issues as they unfold, including and hearing all individuals involved. Special attention must be paid to preserving roles and observing the needs for modifications of roles.

Preparation for the handling of patient flow, phone calls, and refills once EMR has gone live must be done at least 2 months in advance. One month prior to going live there should be an opportunity for everyone who will be using the system to play with the software, to use it, and become familiar with it prior to using it at the point of care. At the time of going live, there should be lots of support from information support services. Patients should be informed about the transition. Be proactive at every step. Build an esprit de corps. While this will not be a panacea, it can be a positive experience for everyone. Keeping in mind, always, the ultimate goal is improved care for our patients.

Chapter 3
Selecting an EMR

Kenneth G. Adler

In a time of drastic change it is the learners who inherit the future. The learned usually find themselves equipped to live in a world that no longer exists
— Eric Hoffer, American social writer and philosopher

Abstract With over 200 EMR products to choose from, selecting an EMR for a practice can be an overwhelming task. The author, Kenneth Adler, MD, MMM, a widely published EMR expert, makes this complex process clear. This chapter outlines the key questions you should ask yourself regarding your motivations, resources, and expectations and then describes a logical 12-step process you can follow to help you make the best selection possible. The recommended steps are as follows: Identify your decision makers, Clarify your goals, Research your options, Establish your requirements, Narrow your options, Attend demonstrations, Check references, Rank the vendors, Conduct site visits, Select a finalist, Solidify organizational commitment, and Negotiate a contract. Each step is described with plenty of practical detail and helpful suggestions. In addition, Dr. Adler provides useful tips on how practice management systems figure into the selection process, EMR certification, reputable information sources, consultants, EMR usability, and more.

Keywords EHR Selection · EMR Selection · Choosing an EHR · How to choose an EHR · EHR Vendors · EHR Site Visits · EHR Ratings · EHR Demonstrations · EHR Certification · EHR Usability · Kenneth Adler · CCHIT · EHR Consultants · EHR User Satisfaction Surveys · Electronic Medical Records · Electronic Health Records

K.G. Adler (✉)
Independent Health IT Consultant and Practicing Family Physician, Adler Health IT Consulting and Arizona Community Physicians, 5300 East Erickson St. Suite 108, Tucson, AZ 85712, USA
e-mail: kadler@azacp.com

N.S. Skolnik (ed.), *Electronic Medical Records*, Current Clinical Practice,
DOI 10.1007/978-1-60761-606-1_3, © Springer Science+Business Media, LLC 2011

Introduction

Many physicians have difficulty in figuring out where to start once they have decided to choose an EMR for their office. With over 200 products to choose from, it is easy to become overwhelmed and fears over the risk of choosing the wrong product can become immobilizing. How do you pick a product that will best suit your needs when you are not sure what your needs are? How do you pick a company that will continue to improve its product's functionality and stay current with the latest standards in health information technology? You realize that this is a huge long-term commitment and that if you make a poor decision you could put the lifeblood of your practice, your medical records, in jeopardy. As of the time of this book's publication, EMR products have proprietary programming and databases and are not significantly interoperable. Once you commit to a product, it will be very difficult and expensive to change to another one down the road. With over 200 companies making EMRs, will the company you pick survive? No one wants to buy a "mission critical" product from a company that might not be in business in 5 years.

The purpose of this chapter is to help you navigate the minefield of EMR selection with a rational plan and confidence. If you are willing to invest reasonable effort in the process, the job of choosing an EMR need not be overwhelming, and you can confidently reduce your risk of making a regrettable decision. With the right attitude, the process might even be fun.

Questions to Ask Yourself

Question One: Why Do I Want to Do This?

This is the first and most important question you should ask yourself. The following qualify as good answers:

- To improve the quality of the care I provide
- To improve my operational efficiency
- To improve my customer service level
- To be able to e-prescribe
- To qualify as a "Patient-Centered Medical Home"
- To be able to do "Pay for Performance"

An acceptable answer but the one that is not sufficient in itself is:

- To qualify for ARRA (American Recovery and Reinvestment Act of 2009) stimulus dollars

Poor answers are:

- Because everyone else is doing it
- I don't know

Being able to answer this first question will help you focus on what matters. It will provide a rationale for you to keep going if and when the going gets tough. All the good answers listed above CAN be accomplished with an EMR – IF you choose one that is appropriate for YOU and IF you implement it well (but let us save that for the next chapter).

Question Two: "Does My Practice Have the Technical Skill and Resources to Manage an EMR by Itself?"

The answer to this question will allow you to determine if you need to outsource some, nearly all, or all of the technical aspects of running an EMR. Once you convert your paper charts to electronic charts, your practice data will be far more accessible and useful in many ways. The negative side of that is that computer systems are at risk for having "downtime" and electronic data is at risk for corruption and even catastrophic loss. You will need to ensure that your EMR rarely goes "down," that it maintains its speed and stability, and finally that if a catastrophe occurs, you have a disaster recovery plan that will work.

Based on the answer to the above question, you will need to decide if you want to host your own servers on-site, host them but have a professional computer service manage them for you, or have everything managed for you off-site. Services that allow you to outsource everything are called ASPs (Application Service Providers) or SaaS (Software as a Service). The company making the product, or a delegated company, manages your program and data for you in a data center. You only need a high-speed internet connection, end-user computers (desktops, laptops, and/or tablets), printers, and a scanner. This type of service is offered on a monthly sub-scription basis per provider and should offer you ownership of your data and a way to retrieve it if your contract should expire or if the company goes bankrupt. In SaaS you will have a Service Level Agreement (SLA) which should clearly state your data ownership rights as well as the degree of guaranteed "availability" – how much downtime is acceptable before financial penalties against the hosting provider kick in. Ninety-nine percent availability sounds good, but it is not. It means that 1% of the time your EMR could be unavailable to you. That equates to 101 minutes (1.7 hours) per week. Imagine trying to efficiently run an office when you cannot access any records, exchange any electronic messages with the staff, or make any appoint-ments for 1.7 unpredictable hours during a busy office schedule every week. If you are lucky, maybe the downtime will only occur at night. And that downtime guaran-tee only applies to failures that your EMR company can control. If your high-speed internet connection goes down for 5 hours on a busy Monday, the internet provider is not going to pay you for your lost productivity that day.

Given the above scenarios, some doctors feel more comfortable not being depen-dent on the wiles of an internet connection or a remote host. They like the idea of having physical ownership of their servers and data. But you have to ask your-self if that sense of security is illusory. Are you going to do as good a job as a company with trained professionals and the resources to maintain elaborate backup systems? A compromise position is to own the servers yourself, but have someone else manage them for you.

Question Three: What Is My Tolerance for Risk?

Are you the sort of person who buys more insurance than others? Do you get anxious at the thought of things not going exactly as planned? If so, then you can narrow your choices in the EMR world dramatically. You will want a relatively large EMR company with a sizable market share and proven track record that has been around longer than most of its competitors. This will likely limit your choice to less than ten products. You will also pay more for that security. On the other hand if you are willing to go with a product from a lesser known and relatively new company you will have many more options. You may find a great product at a great price from a company that provides great service. But you will also increase your risk of buying a product from a vendor that will be purchased by another vendor, or worse, go out of business.

Question Four: Do I Need a Kia or a Lexus?

You might want a Lexus but do you really need one? You may well have very legitimate reasons for needing a fancier, more expensive product in your practice. If you buy an inexpensive product that reduces your productivity, that is false economy. You cannot and should not focus solely on the cost of the product. That is a common error for those choosing an EMR. Your biggest "cost" is how much the product can enhance your productivity and reduce your costs – or not. Currently most EMRs will do a better job of reducing costs (e.g., eliminating transcription costs, paper costs, staff hours, etc.) than increasing provider productivity (e.g., allowing you to see more patients in the same amount of time). But cost reduction clearly goes to the bottom line and will be an important consideration for many.

Some of the more expensive products are designed for multi-site practices with multiple specialties. If you are a solo practitioner in one site, you will not want that degree of complexity, so why pay for it? Some products offer more features than others. So you need to know what features are important to you. Finally some products accomplish a certain function like e-prescribing faster (with fewer mouse clicks) than others. You might want to pay for that.

A 12-Step Program

A rational, considered, and comprehensive approach to EMR selection is necessary in order to have a successful outcome. The 12 steps outlined below can be used for almost any business-critical software purchase. I would like to say that choosing an

EMR is easy and that the cost of making a mistake is low. Unfortunately, at this writing, EMRs are not standardized commodities and the cost of making a poor decision is definitely high, so a clear, well thought-out approach is important [1].

Step 1: Identify Your Decision Makers

A common mistake in EMR selection is for one of the leaders in a practice, such as a managing partner or an office manager, to go pretty far down the selection road before involving others. They may well end up selecting a product that meets their needs or many of the staff's needs, but it is likely that they will overlook one or more functions that are important to others in the practice.

Even if this person has deep personal knowledge of everyone's work – from the receptionists to medical assistants to physicians – and even if this person has outstanding instincts and follows the 12 steps outlined here this is still a bad approach.

Why? Well, it has to do with managing change. An EMR represents a very large change to an office that has always used paper records. Everyone's work is affected. How people accomplish task (called "workflow" in the management and software worlds) changes. New tasks will appear and old ones disappear. People have to learn new skills. It is unsettling to many, and resistance to change is the rule. A few influential people who are unhappy about all this change, and who feel it was imposed on them unreasonably, can easily derail the whole process.

You see, selection of an EMR is hard, but implementation is even harder. Choosing the right product for your practice is not enough. Involving the right people in the selection process helps minimize the chance of failure later during implementation. Communicating with everyone else in the practice will be important too. So who should be on your selection team? Since EMRs affect clinical processes so much, a respected, influential physician should lead or at least co-lead the selection process. In the parlance of EMR vendors, lead physicians involved in the selection and implementation of EMRs are commonly called "physician champions." The team also needs a senior manager, who will be the office manager in nearly all cases. Besides the office manager and physician champion, it is wise to involve an influential representative from your back-office and one from your front office. If you have more than three physicians in your practice, I would recommend that at least two physicians be involved.

If you are in a smaller practice, your selection committee will most likely be the group that makes the decision about the actual purchase. If you are a solo physician, undoubtedly you will be the ultimate decider. Yet you will be wise to listen carefully to the recommendations of others on your "committee." If you are in a large practice, your selection committee may report to a Board and/or Chief Executive that will ultimately make the final decision. In that case, the selection committee should keep that board or person regularly informed about their process and activities as things proceed.

Step 2: Clarify Your Goals

Although it might seem obvious and perhaps unnecessary, this is the time to sit down with your committee and formally declare what you as a practice hope to accomplish by purchasing and implementing an EMR. This is actually a critical step and should make the steps that follow easier. To quote Yogi Berra, "If you don't know where you are going, you might not get there."

This step brings us back to Question 1. Go over those bulleted points with your selection team. Prioritize your goals. As the selection process proceeds, your goals list will help you focus on the features of EMRs that really matter to you. Keep referring back to it.

Another way to elucidate your goals is to ask yourselves what your practice does well? What would you like to do better? Where are your inefficiencies and where are your revenue opportunities? This is a good time to be self critical, or to bring in outside help to look at your practice with a fresh perspective. But remember, an EMR is only a tool, not a panacea. It may be able to help you in the areas that matter most to you, but perhaps the answer lies elsewhere.

Step 3: Research Your Options

A lot of information is available about EMRs – perhaps too much. This makes it confusing to know what information to seek out and rely on. Here is a strategy that can help you focus your learning experience. I will outline the steps and in subsequent paragraphs give you more detail.

First, gain a general understanding of what EMRs are and what they can and cannot do. Reading this book is a good start. Second, learn what specific functionality is available in EMRs and which functionality is most important to you. Third, decide whether you plan to keep your current practice management system (PMS) or whether you plan to get a new one. Fourth, decide what type of certification you require your EMR to have. Remember, in order to qualify for stimulus dollars your EMR must meet the meaningful use criteria outlined in Chapter 1, and certification is one way that will be available to help ensure that your EMR meets those criteria. Fifth, identify whether you are a small practice (generally 1–3 providers, i.e., physicians and advanced level practitioners), medium practice (roughly 3–20 providers), large practice (20–100 providers), or a very large practice (100 + providers.) Sixth, decide whether you want to go with an ASP or SaaS service (more on that follows). Finally, come up with a preliminary list of EMR candidates – ones that will either interface with your PMS or come as an integrated EMR–PMS, have the certification you are looking for, and are commonly utilized by practices of your size.

If you apply these filters to over 200 EMR products out there you will likely come up with a preliminary list of 15–30 candidate EMRs.

What Practice Management System Are You Going to Use?

If you are happy with your current PMS and expect that it will serve the needs of your practice for many years to come, you will likely decide to keep it and thus choose an EMR that will work with it. This is critical. You do not want your staff to have to enter demographic and appointment data twice so the two systems need to be able to communicate with each other. On the other hand, if you are not thrilled about your PMS or think it has outlived its usefulness, you will want to look at "integrated EMRs" – EMRs that are packaged with a PMS and where both work off the same database. The advantage of an integrated product is that you will not have to deal with an electronic interface that can potentially introduce errors, and since you are working off of one database, reporting should be easier. Theoretically the product may be faster. The drawback of course is that although you may love the EMR portion, you might not care as much for the PMS portion. And of course a good PMS is a critical component in the financial success of your practice. In addition, if you like your PMS, the cost of an EMR alone should be less than that of an integrated product.

If you decide to keep your PMS, you should ask that vendor which EMRs they have done interfaces with and with whom they've had the best working relationships. Conversely if you ask the EMR vendor which PMS they can interface with, they will likely reply, not wanting to disappoint you, "all of them."

Understanding Certification

As this book is being written, major changes are incurring in EMR certification. Through 2009, the only game in town has been the Certification Commission for Health Information Technology (CCHIT). They have been certifying products since 2006. Each year their certification criteria have gotten tougher. Their certification is based on functionality and prospective candidates have to go through several highly structured clinical scenarios with their products and pass all steps to become certified. In 2006, 56 products met their criteria while in 2007 it was 53 and in 2008 75 products received certification. You will not find any CCHIT certifications for 2009 and 2010 because in late 2009, CCHIT started their "CCHIT Certified 2011 Ambulatory EHR" certification process in response to the HITECH legislation from the ARRA of 2009.

In addition, at the time of writing this chapter, two groups – CCHIT and the Drummond Group – have indicated that they will apply to be certifiers under the CMS program legislated by HITECH (ARRA) (see Chapter 1). This is a more focused certification, showing that EMRs can perform with "meaningful use." That means that they will be able to do electronic ordering like e-prescribing, create quality of care reports, and be able to exchange information electronically with other systems. The details of this certification were finalized in July 2010.

Certainly you will want your product to have CMS certification so you can potentially receive ARRA dollars, but you may also want your product to have full CCHIT certification to reassure yourself that it is a fully functional product.

More About ASPs/SaaS

If at this point you are thinking that you want to host your own servers, it is worth pointing out even more explicitly that it takes a lot of technical expertise to safely and successfully manage mission critical software. You need to have the right type of hardware (servers, hubs, routers, backup device(s), etc.) in addition to end-user PCs/tablets/notebooks, printers, scanners, etc. You need a safe environment for your servers, e.g., physically secure, temperature-controlled, and fire-suppressant ready, with an uninterruptible power supply. You need to have someone who can troubleshoot and correct problems quickly when they occur, someone to do routine server maintenance, someone who can correct interface error messages on a daily basis, someone who will manage daily data backups, and someone who knows how to test upgrades and patches to your software prior to putting them in the live environment. If you are lucky, you might even be able to find one person who can do all that. Alternatively, you can have your own servers and hire a technology support service to do this for you. That is what many small practices with their own servers do. Typically only much larger practices can afford to have all their technology needs served by in-house staff.

So at first blush, the ASP/SaaS sounds easy and more desirable than the do-it-yourself approach. Not only are you delegating the technical stuff to professionals who take a lot of responsibility off your shoulders, but the start-up costs are much less. However long term costs of a subscription model can easily outpace the do-it-yourself approach if you can manage that well.

Another potential concern with ASPs (now more commonly called SaaS) is that application speed historically has been slower with them, but that is improving. Not uncommonly in ASP EMRs, individual application pages have been known to take from 1 to 4 seconds to load from a remote server. As a busy clinician, you will want to see those page load times at 1 second or less.

How can that issue be ameliorated? In the case of application speed, request a guaranteed average page load time from your vendor in your SLA. On your end you can improve your application speed by spending money on a dedicated high-speed internet connection – typically a T1 line. Since you will need a continuous internet connection, and because local internet connections occasionally go down, you should seriously consider investing in a second (redundant) internet connection as well.

Information Sources

Remember, your goal in the current step, *Step 3: Research Your Options,* is to learn about EMRs – to have the background knowledge that you can then apply in *Step 4:*

Establish Your Requirements so you can come up with a preliminary list of EMR candidates in *Step 5: Narrow Your Options.* The following are all good potential sources of information: books, specialty-sponsored EMR information, EMR consultants, trade shows, EMR user-satisfaction surveys and ratings reports, and do-it-yourself web surfing with a focus on EMR selection websites. The last option of course is the cheapest. Let us take these in turn.

Books

There are a number of books on EMRs but most do not focus on selection. Besides this book, you can find books on EMRs from the Health Information and Management Systems Society (HIMSS), www.himss.org, and from the American Health Information Management Association (AHIMA), www.ahima.org, and medical societies like the AMA, www.ama-assn.org.

Specialty-Sponsored EMR Information

The three main primary care specialty societies offer useful EHR information sites to their members. The American Academy of Family Physicians (AAFP) offers the *Center for Health Information Technology* at www.centerforhit.org. This is an outstanding site with a wealth of information that is open to all. In addition it offers reviews of over 90 EMRs and an EMR E-mail discussion list for AAFP members only. The American College of Physicians (ACP) has a lot of useful information on EMRs and HIT at www.acponline.org/running_practice/technology. This includes an EHR Partners Program that allows ACP members to compare 22 CCHIT certified products. Most of the information on the ACP site is only available to ACP members. The American Academy of Pediatrics (AAP) has posted reviews of over 30 EMRs at www.aapcocit.org/emr that is accessible to all. Additionally, for AAP members only, the site has a contact list of fellow pediatricians using EMRs listed by product and state.

EMR Consultants

If you do not want to be bothered by doing a lot of research on EMRs and are willing to spend money to avoid that responsibility, you can hire a consultant. There are a lot of self-designated EMR consultants out there, but unfortunately there is no generally accepted credentialing process for them. Pretty much anyone can call themselves a consultant. That being said, there are a number of knowledgeable and experienced consultants out there. Here is a link to a list of some of the better known consultants: www.providersedge.com/ehr_links_consulting_firms.htm

Trade Shows

From the mid 1980s to the mid 2000s, the annual *Towards an Electronic Patient Record (TEPR)* conference was the place to go to see all the different EMR vendors in action. The final TEPR show was held in 2009. The conference where you can currently visit the most EMR vendors at once, and have lots of formal educational opportunities on health information technology as well, is the annual *Health Information and Management Systems Society (HIMSS)* conference. In addition numerous CME venues, both regional and national, use EMR vendors as sponsors, and thus offer the opportunity to view a more limited number of EMR vendors at one time.

EMR Ratings and User Satisfaction Surveys

Three sources in particular offer useful EMR ratings and user satisfaction surveys. The AC Group, www.acgroup.org, offers an annually updated, very comprehensive comparison ranking of EMR vendors based on over 4000 EMR and PMS functions and 40 company viability features. It segregates vendors by the practice sizes they serve. It can be purchased online for less than $100. KLAS, www.klasresearch.com, is a healthcare software technology ranking company. It annually researches and ranks EMR vendors by targeted practice size and is a well respected organization. Unfortunately their reports are expensive, running in the hundreds of dollars. Family Practice Management, a practice management journal sponsored by the AAFP, has been publishing EMR user satisfaction survey results every 2 years since 2005. Their 2009 survey [2], www.aafp.org/fpm, features user satisfaction results from 2012 family physicians using 142 different systems. The report focuses on a comparison of the 20 most popular systems, the systems used by 84 percent of the respondents.

Web Sites

If you search the internet only using the term *EMR* or *Electronic Medical Record* you may miss a number of useful sites. Many authors and sites use the term *EHR* or *Electronic Health Record* instead. Some authors and organizations make semantic distinctions between the two terms, but many do not. Interestingly both the government (HITECH legislation) and CCHIT use the term EHR in place of EMR. So at the time of this book's publication, you will want to search using both terms or acronyms in order not to miss any useful sites.

A useful starting place is a web site that offers links in one place to numerous EMR vendors. One such site is EHRscope, www.ehrscope.com/emr-comparison, which offers links to over 250 EMR products and allows you to filter EMRs on the criteria I mentioned above, thus allowing you to quickly narrow in on products that will be most relevant for you. Users of the site should be aware that it is a commercial site with sponsorship by Nuance, the makers of Dragon Medical, the most popular speech recognition software used in conjunction with EMRs.

Another useful EMR information and search site is www.EMRupdate.com. The site claims to be unbiased and independent but it receives sponsorship from several major EMR vendors. In addition, as of 2010, its blog appears to be dominated by individuals with economic ties to various vendors.

Step 4: Establish Your Requirements

Consider this scenario. One physician thinks an EMR will help them code at a higher level and make more money. Another physician wants to be able to access their charts from home. A nurse practitioner really wants to have more accurate and dynamic problem lists and be able to improve the patient education he or she provides. A medical assistant wants to reduce or eliminate annoying calls from pharmacies asking for clarification. Another medical assistant simply wants to eliminate "lost charts" and the time it takes to get access to a chart so she can return a phone call. An office manager wants to be able to do pay for performance reporting and to be able to create a wide variety of reports easily on an ad hoc basis. A records person would like to be able to batch e-fax reports from a chart to a consultant and they would like to be able to download an entire large patient chart to a CD to give to a patient rather than having to waste time and money printing hundreds of pages.

Can all these goals be accomplished with an EMR? Certainly. Do all EMRs do all of these things? No. Do the EMRs that do all of these things equally well? Almost certainly not. Some help you work more efficiently than others. Some do reporting much better than others. Some are slick at e-prescribing, others are not.

At this stage in the game, your EMR selection team should sit down and list your EMR functionality needs in three prioritized categories: (1) must-have functions, (2) would like to have functions, and (3) optional functions.

RFP/RFI

In the past I had advised readers to undertake the ponderous task of writing a request for proposal (RFP), a document that tells prospective vendors about a client and its resources and requests specific answers to numerous detailed questions about a vendor and its product or service. RFPs allow for side by side comparisons of different vendors and are particularly useful for a service or product that is not standardized, where a lot of customization is expected. Over the last few years EMRs have become much more standardized, and a lot more information is readily available about them. With the exception of very large medical groups, I no longer recommend RFPs. In its place I recommend that all practices, even solo practices, create a short Request For Information (RFI) document. After you have done your research, you will submit this document to vendors that interest you , in order to get even more detailed information than you have been able to get from the information sources listed in Step 3.

What should be in an RFI? First you will describe yourself – your practice size, your current practice software, hardware, network, and internet infrastructure. Then you will list your established requirements – the must haves and like to haves. Then you will ask for vendor information – in the form of product brochures and financial reports and in the form of specific questions important to you that you do not think will be available in brochures. You should be sure to ask the vendor details about itself – company history, particularly with regard to their EMR product, and for their financial statistics. A company's financial stability will be very important to you, as the purchase of an EMR will initiate a long-term partnership between you and the vendor. This is a relationship that, once formed, will be costly to sever. You should inquire about the number of practices that are actively using their product nationally, in your state, and in your specialty as well as the breakdown in the size of those practices. You will also want to get ballpark information about costs, as well as information about their implementation services, training, and support. You should state who the key contact person in your practice is and any deadlines that you have. This RFI document can be as short as two pages, compared to an RFP which commonly runs dozens of pages long.

Step 5: Narrow Your Options

OK, so now you have an idea what is out there, which products are highly rated, and what your needs are. You have applied your "filters" to over 200 products out there, perhaps using EHRscope and have come up with a list of 15 products. You then sent out an RFI to those 15 products and now your selection "committee" has narrowed your options down to 5 products or so. It is now time to see those products in action.

Step 6: Attend Demonstrations

When you have determined that a product meets all of your specifications on paper, it is time to see it in action. You will ask the vendors to do a demo for you. Ideally this will be done in person but it may be done via the Internet. Typically vendors will offer to do canned scenarios that put their product in the best possible light. You should be aware that the vendor will also be running the product in an "unnatural" environment, i.e., off a server with no competing users or even directly off a laptop with a tiny database to draw on. This may make the product seem faster than it would be in a real working environment, so you will want to investigate that in *Step 9: Conduct Site Visits.*

Optimally you should do two things to make these demos particularly useful. You should ask all vendors who demo for you to run through a standardized script of workflows that you write yourself, and you should have a formal rating tool that all demo attendees individually fill out immediately after the demo. Also do not just invite your clinicians to view the demo. Ask a back office staff member (e.g., medical assistant), your office manager, and perhaps a front office staff member to all demos. They will be looking at the EMR's functionality differently than the clinicians, since their workflows are so different.

The standardized script should not be too hard to create. Think of the tasks that you do commonly and list those. Example should include refilling medications, prescribing new medications, reviewing lab work, answering phone messages, documenting a visit, filling out a problem list, and reviewing prior notes and studies. For the documentation piece, give the vendor a common clinical scenario of a patient coming to the office with multiple medical problems, as vendors will demo a patient with just one straightforward problem, a scenario that is actually uncommon in most of our offices. The tendency of many physicians first looking at EMRs is to focus on the documentation piece. They see the EMR mainly as an electronic way to write notes – but it is much, much more than that. It is an entire electronic solution for your entire office – an intra-office messaging system, task manager, ordering system, e-prescriber and scanned document repository. It is a potential way to exchange information electronically with patients and other physicians. It is a disease management and health maintenance tool as well as a tracking tool for tests not done. It can be a patient education aide and clinical decision support tool as well. What you do not want it to be is an impediment, something that slows you down without adding value.

CCHIT has standardized scripts that ask EMRs to do all the above things. They are available for anyone to see and copy from their website at www.cchit.org/get_certified/open_ambulatory. You can use these scripts yourself or modify them. Just because the vendor's product had to perform these scripts to become certified, doesn't mean that they had to perform them well. I can tell you from my experience as a juror for CCHIT that two products often perform the same function quite differently. One can do it with just a few clicks and in an intuitive way, while another product can do it in a very awkward and time-consuming way. You will need to see several products running through the same script to get a feel for that. Send your test script to the vendor several days to a week before the scheduled demo. You may be tempted to spring it on them, but it is a reasonable courtesy to give them fair warning. That way they can include it, but also show you other things that they think are important about their product. It will also help them budget their time.

A typical demo, if it is reasonably thorough, will take 2–3 hours. That is why, unless you have unlimited time, you will likely want to limit your demos to no more than 5 or so. You should create a rating form for the demo which grades how efficiently and intuitively the product performs the items on your test scripts. That way you can compare your ratings later. It is amazing how after the fourth or fifth demo things start to blur and your memory becomes less clear about what product did what in which way. You may even want to use a formal usability rating scale which we will now discuss.

Usability

Up until recently, usability has been an ignored facet of EMR evaluations. Formal research on software and web page usability has been conducted and some standard principles have been established. Validated usability scales have also been created. Agreed upon usability principles include simplicity, naturalness, consistency, minimizing cognitive overload, efficient interactions, forgiveness and feedback, effective use of language, effective information presentation, and preservation of context [3].

As of its Certified 2011 Ambulatory EHR certification, CCHIT will be conducting usability testing on EMRs utilizing 3 different usability scales and then combing the scores into a single ranking of 1–5. At this time vendors will have the option of allowing their scores to be published or not. Hopefully in the future, that will become mandatory. These scales can be found at www.cchit.org/get_certified/open_ambulatory.

Step 7: Check References

Check at least three references for each vendor that remains in the running at this point. Try to gather several perspectives from each reference site – a physician, IT manager, and office manager would be ideal. Each looks at the EHR differently. The physician focuses on functionality, the IT person on technical features, and the manager on the quality of vendor service, training, and cost. Peer to peer interviews are best; ideally those respective roles in your practice will talk to their colleagues at the reference site.

Your vendor will offer you a list of references. These will be their most satisfied customers and they may even receive some form of compensation, such as discounts on the software, for talking to you. Keep that bias in mind, but go ahead and talk to them anyway. My experience is that even at these sites, people can be remarkably frank. Moreover, if these references are not pretty enthusiastic about the product, be concerned. Be sure to ask to speak with reference sites that are similar in practice size and specialty make-up to your own.

Beyond references provided by the vendor, seek out references from sites that were not recommended, ideally sites in your own region or state. Consider going online and trying to tap into user group sites. Be aware, however, that many of these sites are likely to be closed to non-users.

Work from a written check list of questions and write down the responses. You will be using these responses in the next step – ranking the vendors. I would recommend the following questions at a minimum.

Primary questions:

- Overall, how satisfied are you with this product?
- If you could choose an EMR again, would you choose this one?
- Do you think this product is good value? Too expensive or priced fairly?
- Are you happy with the support provided by your vendor?

- Are you happy with the training provided by your vendor?
- How easy and intuitive is this product to use?
- Are you satisfied with the product's speed? If not, why not?
- Is there anything you would like to see changed about the product?

Secondary questions:

- Are you happy with the e-prescribing functionality?
- Are you happy with the documentation functionality?
- Are you happy with the disease and health management functionality?
- Are you happy with the reports it can produce?
- Do you have any lab, hospital, or radiology interfaces? Which? How well do they work?

For all these questions, if the answer is not unequivocally positive, ask follow-up questions to find out why.

Step 8: Rank the Vendors

Before you can do an overall ranking of your remaining vendors you will need to do one more piece of data collection and analysis. You need to rank the remaining vendors by cost. This can be tricky. Vendors do not present costs in a uniform fashion. All costs are not explicit. I recommend adding up purchase, implementation, and maintenance costs and amortizing them over 5 years. Then compare total first 5 year costs. You will need to collect data on the following items for each vendor so you can compare costs on an apples-to-apples basis.

Purchase costs:

- EMR software
- Hardware – server, routers, switches, backup, PCs, printers, scanners, etc.
- Other software – e.g., user licenses for required applications
- Interfaces
- Network upgrades

Implementation costs:

- Implementation fees (if not included in initial software cost)
- Training

Maintenance costs:

- Software (upgrades and support)
- Interfaces
- IT staff related
- Network/bandwidth

Add these all up for each vendor and rank them with the lowest cost vendor ranked as 1, the next as 2, and so forth.

You will now want to get your committee together and rank the products next by functionality and usability. I recommend that each person in your selection group do their own rankings first – listing in order the product they think is best, then second best, and so on. Then you will need to discuss your individual rankings and come to a consensus ranking. The ranking should be based primarily on the results of Step 6, the demonstrations, but can be supplemented by information you gained from the reference calls as well as your research in Step 3. If you quantified your demonstration rankings, scoring each vendor, this step may already be largely completed. You will still want to discuss the final rankings in light of what you have learned about the product outside the demos.

Next you will want each selection committee member to rank the vendor based on "vendor characteristics" such as quality of support, quality of training, financial strength of the company, and vendor "reputation." This information will largely come from your reference calls.

Now you are ready to combine these three rankings into one overall ranking. You need to decide how you want to weight these three factors. The natural tendency of clinicians is to want to give the bulk of the weighting to functionality and usability, the second most to cost and the least to vendor characteristics. This is a bad idea. How well your vendor delivers on service and training and whether your vendor will still be in business in 5 years will become very important to you once you implement the EMR. Functionality typically improves more over time than vendor characteristics. Moreover if you use cost as your primary criteria, you may end up sorely disappointed and actually lose money. The largest financial impact of the EMR will not be the initial investment cost, but rather its financial impact on productivity and cost savings in the long run. The phrase "you get what you pay for" more likely than not applies here.

The weighting my office used when we did this was 40% for functionality/usability, 40% for vendor characteristics, and 20% for cost.

A visual representation of a sample ranking process is as follows:

| Component | Vendors | | | | | | | |
| | Rankings | | | | | | | |
	A Raw	A Weighted	B Raw	B Weighted	C Raw	C Weighted	D Raw	D Weighted
Functionality and usability	1	0.4	2	0.8	4	1.6	3	1.2
Vendor characteristics	2	0.8	4	1.6	3	1.2	1	0.4
Cost	2	0.4	1	0.2	3	0.6	4	0.8
Total	**5**	**1.6**	**7**	**2.6**	**10**	**3.4**	**8**	**2.4**

Here the weighting is:

Functionality/Usability 40%; Vendor Characteristics 40%; Cost 20%

Here the raw ranking is:

Vendor A
Vendor B
Vendor D
Vendor C

But the weighted ranking is:

Vendor A
Vendor D
Vendor B
Vendor C

Note that with the weighted score, Vendor D moves from third place to second place. Vendor A with the lowest total weighted ranked score wins!

Step 9: Conduct Site Visits

Why wait until this late in the selection process to do site visits? First, a site visit is best used as a confirmatory step, not an initial information gathering step. Site visits are usually too costly and too time consuming to do a lot of them (unless you can do them in your own community). So you will want to know as much as possible about the products you are interested in before going to visit a site where they are in use. The purpose of the site visit is to see if the EMR works as promised in the "live environment." You may only want to do site visits for your top two choices. If the products do not perform as expected, you may need to go back to Step 8 and redo it.

Who should you bring on a site visit? Ideally you would bring a clinician, a back-office person, an administrator, and an IT person. Each one should shadow and meet with a colleague in their respective area.

Step 10: Select a Finalist

If there were no big surprises on your site visit, you can now formally identify your top choice. It is important strategically to identify a backup choice as well. This gives you more leverage in the negotiation process. You should let both vendors know that they are your top two choices. This sets up a potential competition that will hopefully lead to better pricing and contract terms for you. Do not lie and tell your second choice that they are your first choice if they are not, but let them know that they are still in the running. You can let your first choice know that they are your preferred choice, but make sure you let them know nicely that you are willing to walk away if the two of you cannot achieve an acceptable price and contract.

Step 11: Solidify Organizational Commitment

You have one more thing to do before you negotiate the contract. You need to go back to the rest of your practice that has not been involved in the selection process and bring them up to date. Hopefully they have been receiving communication from you about this process all along. It is a great idea to have the vendor gives a demonstration of their product to your entire staff. You should encourage questions. Hopefully no one will ask questions that you have not already addressed. But if someone raises an important concern that you had not considered, you should maintain the flexibility to reevaluate your ranking and even go back to gather more information if needed.

Even if you have been very thorough and anticipated and addressed every concern and question prior to this all-staff demo, this demo still has merit. It helps give everyone a sense of involvement and ownership in the process (especially if it is not presented as a fait accompli). Staff involvement is an important part of the change management process. Anyone involved in implementing an EMR should have a good understanding of change management. A classic and readable book on that topic is a book by John Kotter called *Leading Change* [4].

Step 12: Negotiate a Contract

You may end up only negotiating one or two or perhaps a handful of major software contracts in your career. The EMR vendor you will negotiate with does them all the time. Hire a lawyer to help you with this step. This is such an important purchase for you that you do not want to overlook something or commit to something that you will regret later. You should hire a legal counsel with substantial experience in software contracting.

Here are some key issues to consider:

Contract Duration – Be sure to clarify the contract duration. If it is not a lifetime contract, then what happens when the contract term expires?

Ownership Transferability – Be sure to clarify the license scope, Is it transferrable? Obviously that is something you will want if you are ever in a position to sell your practice and retire. What happens if the vendor ceases to exist? How will you be able to transfer your practice data to a new EMR if you need to in the future? Since proprietary software is non-standard an IT expert would not be able to convert your data to a new system without understanding the data base schema and the software source code. One way to handle that contractually is to have the vendor put their source code in escrow in the case of bankruptcy or dissolution.

ICD-10 Compliance – Will your product achieve compliance with the planned federally mandated change from ICD-9 coding to ICD-10 coding? Make sure that they guarantee they will be in your contract.

ARRA Certification – Will your EMR achieve and maintain ARRA certification. You should seek such a guarantee in your contract to ensure that you will be a candidate to apply for stimulus funding.

Price – Finally and perhaps most important, ask for a discount! Prices of EMRs and terms of payment are clearly negotiable.

Open Source and Free Software

Perhaps you have heard that there is free EMR software out there. There are in fact two types: proprietary free products that are funded by advertisements and open source software. Remember that there is no such thing as a free lunch. Free products are only free in so far as there is no cost for the software itself. Yet typically, EMR software accounts for just 15–25% of the total cost of ownership [5]. The costs you will incur include implementation costs, maintenance costs, hardware costs, interface costs, the costs of any associated commercial software licenses, and the cost of any additional EMR-related personnel.

Proprietary

The best known free proprietary software available at the time of this book's publication is "Practice Fusion." This is available as an easily downloadable program that requires relatively little training. It functions like an ASP. Currently it is not CCHIT certified.

Open Source

A number of open source EMRs exist. Open source means that the source code is available to anyone and can be modified by the user for custom use as they see fit. If you are a programmer that enjoys tinkering, this may be an option you might want to consider. And even if you are not, several products have commercial implementation and support that has grown up around them. The advantage of an open source product is that you do save money by not paying for the software license. However the amount of time you will spend implementing it and customizing it may negate some or all of those savings. Plus as of this writing, open source products have less functionality than proprietary products, especially in the area of e-prescribing and ordering, but that may be changing. From an aesthetic point of view, open source products tend to be less attractive looking since programmers have focused on function rather than appearance.

Here is a list of some open source products:

World Vista EHR – www.worldvista.org
Clear Health – www.clear-health.com
FreeMED – www.freemedsoftware.org (site being moved)
OpenEMR – www.oemr.org

Conclusion

Selecting an EMR is a complex, time consuming endeavor. It is not something to be done impulsively. It requires forethought. Your EMR will have a major impact on your practice. If you carefully follow the steps outlined here, you are far more likely to have a positive outcome. In summary those steps are:

Step 1: Identify your decision makers
Step 2: Clarify your goals
Step 3: Research your options
Step 4: Establish your requirements
Step 5: Narrow your options
Step 6: Attend demonstrations
Step 7: Check references
Step 8: Rank the vendors
Step 9: Conduct site visits
Step 10: Select a finalist
Step 11: Solidify organizational commitment
Step 12: Negotiate a contract

References

1. Adler, KG. *How to Select an Electronic Health Record System*. Fam Pract Manag. 2005; 12(2): 55–62.
2. Edsall, RL, Adler, KG. *The 2009 EHR User Satisfaction Survey: Responses from 2012 Family Physicians*. Fam Pract Manag. 2009; 16(6): 10–16.
3. HIMSS EHR Usability Task Force. *Defining and Testing EMR Usability: Principles and Proposed Methods of EMR Usability Evaluation and Rating*. June 2009.
4. Kotter, JP. *Leading Change*. Boston, MA: Harvard Business School Press; 1996.
5. Terry, K. *An EMR for Free? Just Like Lunch, There's No Such Thing*. Physicians Practice – Technology Guide. June 2008; 15–19.

Chapter 4
Pre-implementation Planning and Workflow Analysis

Christopher Notte

> *The will to win is important, but the will to prepare is vital.*
> – Joe Paterno, Football Coach, Penn State

Abstract This chapter underscores the premise that preparation is the key to success. In the world of HIT, this notion is critical. Avoiding failure when implementing an EHR is dependent on asking the right questions long before taking the first step and continually re-evaluating the answers to those questions along the way. With a focus on teamwork, and a healthy amount of enthusiasm, practices can create buy-in and ownership of the process and ensure employee satisfaction. Ultimately, it is not the limitations of technology that leads to the untimely demise of EHR installations. Instead, failure is caused by impaired office efficiency, frustrated staff, and decreased physician satisfaction resulting from not taking the proper steps to prepare along the way.

Keywords EMR pre-implementation planning · Electronic health records · EHR conversion · EHR efficiency · HER cost-effectiveness · Physician champion · Senior manager · HER team

Deciding which electronic health record to purchase is a tremendous challenge, but is only the beginning of the very time-consuming process of EHR conversion. As mentioned previously, no physician practices alone, and every member of one's practice or health network will be affected by the transition. More importantly, no matter how capable or effective the EHR is, there is no guarantee of success. According to information from the AC Group, a respected healthcare tech research organization (www.acgroup.org), over 70% of EHR implementations fail. This number is staggering and disturbing, and begs the question of why this is the case.

C. Notte (✉)
Doylestown Hospital, 1700 Horizon Drive, Chalfont, PA 18914-3950, USA
e-mail: cmnotte@gmail.com

N.S. Skolnik (ed.), *Electronic Medical Records*, Current Clinical Practice,
DOI 10.1007/978-1-60761-606-1_4, © Springer Science+Business Media, LLC 2011

57

As with any other business decision of this magnitude, adequate preparation is the key to success. Professional athletes know that victory only results from practice, determination, and teamwork. Physicians implementing health information technology (HIT) must accept the same approach and recognize the risks and consequences of failure. This will be an extremely expensive undertaking, and will be made more costly by having to do it more than once.

In this chapter, we'll consider the critical steps necessary to accomplish the conversion process as efficiently and cost-effectively as possible. These should not be novel concepts to anyone who has ever found themselves in a leadership role, as they are widely-accepted strategies for success in any business undertaking. But in the world of healthcare IT, they can be easily disregarded, because many of these concepts can seem to be a distraction from patient care. Ultimately, if the process is successful, the change to an electronic patient record should improve patient care and enhance the satisfaction of both the physician and the patient.

Building the Winning "Transition Team"

The first step toward a successful transition is identifying the principal players and decision-makers who will oversee the implementation of the electronic record. As suggested in the previous chapter, a team may have already been chartered to select and purchase the EHR. At this point, a decision has to be made to determine whether those individuals are the most appropriate to continue in this leadership role. Depending on the size and type of practice, the way in which the "transition team" is structured may look somewhat different from the "selection team." For example, the selection team might comprise senior office staff and care providers, while the transition team may comprise staff members from each department. Regardless, to be effective the team will need strong and influential leadership and diversity in the roles that each of the members play in the practice. A team made up of only physicians is destined for failure, as this unilateral approach will often overlook many of the critical steps necessary for successful and efficient office workflow.

The Physician Champion

When assembling the team, it is essential to establish the "physician champion" who will be responsible for communicating with fellow providers and fostering an attitude of success. This physician need not be someone with tremendous technical ability, though this is certainly helpful. Most importantly, the champion needs to be enthusiastic about the changes that will be occurring and be able to impart that enthusiasm to everyone in the practice. He or she will be able to clearly elucidate and communicate the goals of the HIT implementation, and be available to address any concerns or questions the other physicians may have. Also, this person will have the final word on all decisions that directly affect how care is administered in the exam rooms by the providers.

The choice of "physician champion" may be obvious is some practices, as certain physicians may have a penchant for tech or a strong interest in the success of the roll-out. In solo practices the issue is clearly moot. In many situations, however, the right person to choose may not be initially obvious. Whoever is chosen should be an influential individual with a strong staff rapport. After all, it is much easier for people to get excited about something when they see it promoted by an individual who understands and respects them.

The Senior Manager

The senior manager will be the team member who oversees all aspects of the transition and ensures that the process is moving along on schedule. Most often, this role will fall to the office manager, but may be delegated to another individual if deemed more appropriate. It is critical that the senior manager have a strong grasp on every aspect of office workflow. Also, he or she should have the ability to synthesize many opinions shared by the team into clear and realizable goals. Working hand-in-hand with the physician champion, the manager will cast the vision for the EHR roll-out and be ready to address dissenting concerns.

Throughout the transition process, the senior manager will be responsible for all administrative aspects of the team. This typically entails regular communication with the EHR vendor, serving as go-between for any issues or questions that may arise. He or she may also need to collate and disseminate any documents generated by the team, such as surveys, questionnaires, and requests for information. It will also be the responsibility of the team manager to make sure that realistic goals are established and are consistently re-evaluated, so that at the end all members of the team will feel their needs were addressed.

Moving forward, the senior manager will be a "superuser" of the the EHR, and may share this role with the physician champion. This means both will have advanced training in the operation of all of the available features of the product and may have access to additional functionality. They should be familiar with how every user will employ the new technology so that they can assist them in training and daily operations. Also, they need to ensure that the EHR is operating properly and that users are following the established procedures. For example, they may need to generate queries and/or reports to make sure patient interactions are properly documented and notes are electronically signed.

Selecting the Rest of the Team

Ultimately, the implementation process will be successful only if led by an effective senior manager and physician champion. Once these individuals are identified, their first order of business should be selecting the rest of the team.

The transition team should be a diverse group of individuals from clinical and non-clinical areas. Obviously, in smaller practices, this might mean almost everyone, but in larger offices one representative from each area should be fine. Include both front and back-office staff, as the electronic record will touch every aspect of patient care. It is particularly helpful to choose team members who not only understand the process, but are also enthusiastic about it. A well-chosen team can be the best defense against the inevitable "nay-sayers" who are skeptical about the process!

In multi-doctor groups, having additional care providers on the team can also be very helpful, because these are the individuals responsible for generating income for the practice, and ensuring their ability to work efficiently with the EHR is critical. But take caution against loading the team too heavily with physicians, as it could discourage open dialogue from other staff members and prevent their needs from being fairly addressed. Once the EHR is finally in place, a transition team in which every member feels valued will create the best possibility for long-term physician and staff satisfaction.

Laying Down the Ground Rules

Once the team is selected, an initial meeting should be held to make sure everyone is working from the same playbook. It would be very unusual to find that all of the chosen individuals have a firm understanding of electronic health records. There are typically many misconceptions about health information technology and unrealistic expectations about the process. The team should be clear and in complete agreement with the product that has been chosen, and have access to a demonstration or other resources detailing its functionality. Each member should also know and be comfortable with the reasons why the transition is taking place, as this will be essential when communicating with his or her colleagues and creating buy-in, as we'll discuss this in the next chapter.

A timeline should be laid out for how the team will proceed. Early meetings should focus on "big picture" items, in which the goals that were established when choosing the EHR are re-visited and possibly re-prioritized. Later, the focus should be on analyzing and defining workflow procedures. At each phase, it can be helpful to delegate who will take on each of the various responsibilities. For example, it may make sense for one team member to think about hardware selection, another to examine clinical procedures, and still another to work on coding and billing, etc. When the team meets, each individual can report on their progress and solicit insights from the others. These meetings should occur regularly (i.e., every 2–4 weeks) and will be facilitated by the team manager, who will keep to the schedule and ensure everyone's input is considered.

Soliciting Input and Creating Buy-In

The failures of EHR implementations are often caused by productivity loss, and nothing is more detrimental to productivity than discouraged employees. It is therefore very important to have buy-in from all members of a practice prior to taking the first steps. As stated previously, having influential members in the transition team to help with this can be invaluable.

Early on, a presentation providing an overview of the software can also be very helpful. If the EHR vendor has not already done so, they can often provide a demonstration to the entire office staff highlighting all of the features. This may be the same demo already seen by the selection committee, but at this point it can also be used to address specific questions generated by the transition team. Using an LCD projector in a common area of the office can allow for the inclusion of all the office staff and help to create a sense of comradery.

The next step in creating buy-in from staff is to solicit questions and concerns. It is common for individuals to have anxiety about the transition as it represents a change in their very comfortable routine. Others may be simply "technophobic" and deplore the idea of spending any more time interacting with technology than they already have to. One way to address these issues is to highlight the ways in which the HIT implementation may save time and make life easier. For example, the EHR may avail the possibility of automating appointment reminders and refill requests, simplify the referral process, and increase the legibility of progress notes. What was once unreliably communicated through a myriad of "sticky notes" can now be safely documented in secure electronic communications. Coding and billing can now be optimized to improve charge capture and increase revenue. Time spent on pulling charts will be minimized, while data collection and quality reporting will be dramatically streamlined. There is no process in the office that will not be affected – and hopefully improved – by the EHR. Communicating this in a way that emphasizes the positive aspects of the change, while carefully addressing employee fears and concerns, can build excitement for the transition and ultimately ensure its success.

Workflow Analysis

Few physicians spend time thinking about the "workflow" in their practices, but most would be quick to notice if it were disrupted. Let's face it, we are all creatures of habit, and become comfortable operating within a normal routine. Inevitably, the introduction of health information technology into an office will create a new routine, and there is no question that workflow – and therefore efficiency – will be greatly affected. One way to minimize the disruption is to start with a solid understanding of the current office workflow and identify the key steps essential to maintaining productivity. This begins with asking the right questions and ends with no stone left unturned.

Let's Start at the Very Beginning...

The logical place to begin analyzing workflow is the front desk. This is typically the initial interface between patients and a practice, either in person or through the telephone. Most offices already use computerized practice management tools, so it may be very easy for transition to a full EHR for scheduling patient encounters. Beyond that, however, many physician groups are still relying heavily on paper for intra-office communications. This can be the biggest hurdle to overcome when making the switch.

In all too many practices, staff members jot down sensitive information on "sticky notes" and post them in a place they hope a physician will notice. This is a very dangerous practice on many levels: it provides the opportunity for important messages to be over-looked, does not allow for permanent documentation of critical information, and raises several security and legal issues. With the looming fears of the Health Information Portability and Accountability Act (HIPAA), it is difficult to overstate the concern. Fortunately, the transition to an electronic health record is the ideal time to address this unhealthy practice in the concerted attempt to go "paperless."

One might start by considering simple ergonomics. In order to ditch the sticky notes, the information collected from a phone call needs to be simultaneously and efficiently entered into a computer. This means the staff member will need to type while speaking on the phone, so hands-free headsets may need to be ordered. Also, every employee will need access to a workstation both to send and receive messages.

While at first the simple process of communicating a phone message may seem terribly inefficient with the computer, the eventual time savings can be significant. No longer must an employee engage in furtive searches for patient charts, nor must they track down the doctor to convey the information from the call. A well-implemented EHR should make all the necessary data accessible to the message recipient as soon as he or she logs into the system. If the message is intended for a care provider, that provider can open and review the message even when in the room with another patient, and instantly respond more efficiently than ever before. But this requires a time investment at the outset to develop procedures that the entire staff will follow. If the proper information is not collected consistently, phone calls and other patient interactions can become a logistical nightmare. It therefore makes sense to spend time thinking about how patient information will initially be entered into the electronic record.

In many practices, patients fill out paperwork prior to their initial visit, eliciting past medical history, medications, allergies, and other clinically relevant data. In an attempt to eliminate paper, those same data will now need to be collected electronically. Some offices choose to simply transcribe the information from paper into the EHR. While this may initially be a stopgap solution, it is not an acceptable long-term strategy. For any EHR implementation to be successful, processes should be reduced to as few steps as possible and should not be dependent on paper at all. One way to achieve this is to allow patients to enter data directly into the EHR on their own.

Upon check-in, patients can be handed a notebook or tablet computer, or directed to sit down at a terminal in the waiting room. The computer can prompt them to enter past history and answer questions related to their current visit. This not only collects relevant data, but also can simplify the documentation process for the care provider. It presents some interesting challenges, as well. Once this process is in place, it may preclude certain patients from entering useful information. Patients who are illiterate, physically or mentally challenged, or elderly may find interacting with their physician in this way to be overwhelming or even impossible. Others may be unwilling to use the computer due to perceived security concerns. If the waiting room is not designed to offer privacy, this may mean considering an architectural change, such as installing individual kiosks for patients to sit at for data entry. Regardless of how the technology is employed, the burden will be on the front-office staff to ensure everyone is comfortable using it. This may be time-consuming and ultimately frustrating, so keeping things simple for patients is the key to making it work well.

Moving Patients in the Right Direction

Now that every office task is dependent on the EHR, providers and clinical staff will quickly discover new challenges with electronic documentation. Obviously, a computer is required at every step in the process. This means that everyone will need to carry their own portable PC, or else use stationary workstations available throughout the office.

Many practices find that notebooks or tablets are the least disruptive to existing office workflow, as they take up little space and allow each user to remain "logged in" to just one computer. But even the lightest of notebooks can be cumbersome to carry through an entire patient session, and staff frequently needs both hands free to obtain vital signs or type a chief complaint. It therefore makes sense to provide surfaces for setting the computers down throughout the office. Also, portable computers depend on batteries to keep them running. When considering hardware, opt for computers that allow batteries to be easily swapped and replenished in an external battery charger. There is nothing more frustrating and disruptive to workflow than computer that "dies" suddenly due to a dead battery, resulting in a time-consuming reboot and potential loss of data.

If desktop computers are employed, serious thought must be given to the arrangement of the exam room. The computer should not interfere with the patient encounter. Unlike a portable PC that can be placed on the provider's lap, a workstation sitting on a desk can be a serious obstacle to a face-to-face interaction. Also, some exam rooms are simply too small to allow a permanent workstation to be comfortably integrated into the space. This might make the decision to avoid desktops obvious from the start. But whichever type of computer is employed, the focus should be on seamlessly integrating them into the workflow and avoiding disruptions to the physician–patient relationship.

At this point, another question is who will be responsible to input visit data? Some practices may choose for nursing staff to simply enter vital signs and a chief complaint in preparation for the physician, others may elect for more historical information to be documented before the clinician enters the room. Data entry is time-consuming, so depending on the skill set of the various clinical staff, it may be beneficial to have them do as much of it as possible. Many physicians trust the history obtained by the nurses or medical assistants to become part of the permanent record. Other docs may have staff with more limited clinical experience and only feel comfortable obtaining the history themselves. Whatever rules are established, the process of moving patients through the office must not become an obstacle to efficiency.

The Hand-Off

Once the patient is in the room, the provider must be notified that he or she is ready to be seen. In a paper-based office, there are many ways this might happen: a system of colored flags or lights, a personal notification by the nurse, or merely by the sight of the chart in the rack. While some of these systems may continue once the electronic record is implemented, none take full advantage of the available technology. Most EHR products have built-in functionality which allows for a signal to be sent to the clinician notifying that the patient is ready – some may even offer an audible or visual alert. The hope is that once implemented, the EHR should make the work of communicating a patient's status completely automated.

The software should also allow the care provider to request office services without having to personally track down the staff. During the visit, he or she may decide to order a vaccination, EKG, lab draw, or other office procedure. Hence, the nurse has to be notified, and the EHR should allow for a message to be sent electronically to the appropriate person. Typically, the physician will enter the order into the record, and that order will automatically generate a task for the staff with instructions for what is required. Once received, the staff member will perform the task and document its completion, thereby closing the loop without the need to personally interact with the clinician. At least, this is what should happen if the technology is to be used as designed. It may not be quite this seamless, but thinking through this process in advance and anticipating the road blocks will go a long way toward achieving that goal.

Documenting the Visit

One aspect of electronic health records that doctors fear most is documentation. Whether physicians are used to handwriting or dictating their notes, the new technology will change the way they practice. This is why a great deal of thought should be given to the hardware and input method employed in any EHR installation. As a first step, consider the three basic methods for entering data for the patient encounter:

1. *"Point and click"* – Most EHRs include functionality to minimize typing by offering a "point-and-click" interface for documenting notes. This may be a series of check boxes or drop-down menus through which the clinician makes appropriate selections from pre-set options in the software. Many packages even allow these to be customized, and may allow users to create their own templates and defaults for each chief complaint. This can make writing an encounter note extremely simple.

The computer may use a traditional pointing device, such as a mouse or trackpad, or offer a pen for "tablet" functionality.

While pointing and clicking may at first seem very appealing, it can become quite tiresome if the interface is not user-friendly. In some cases, making the desired selection can mean hunting through multiple options to find it. Not only is this extremely time-consuming, it might lead care providers to choose efficiency over precision. Put differently, choosing from a list encourages one to "settle" on a symptom or description that is not quite exact, in order to minimize the amount of time required to document the note. Compared to dictated or written notes, the end product may not accurately reflect the visit or properly convey the assessment and plan. Specialists intending to use their office notes as correspondence to other physicians may find this ambiguity unacceptable. It may therefore be necessary to consider a more "old-fashioned" approach to documentation.

2. *Free typing* – Physicians have a long reputation for illegible handwriting, and often their typing skills are not much better. It would be unreasonable to think that transitioning to an EHR would have a positive impact on any physician's ability or attitude toward typing. On the contrary, some doctors who are forced to adapt to documenting this way find themselves frustrated and terribly inefficient. To make up for the time loss, they may limit their patient load for a significant period of time. Ultimately, this is unsustainable and will have a dramatic impact on the bottom line.

In contrast, many clinicians may find this method advantageous over others. Some are actually good typists, while others simply find it easier to document precisely. In addition, many EHR products offer built-in capabilities to make typing more efficient, by allowing clinicians to create reusable templates and macros. This avoids the need to repetitively type common verbiage for every visit. The software may even be smart enough to adjust what is "pre-typed" on the note based on the chief complaint. For example, once the provider has selected the reason for the visit, the EHR may automatically populate the note with the symptoms, review of systems, and physical exam findings most commonly entered for that encounter type. Often this can be further customized by provider, so each individual in an office can have their own pre-set language and defaults. Once the clinician begins entering data, he or she simply adds or subtracts information to make the final note complete.

This concept is known as "documentation by exclusion." It encourages more efficient note writing by placing the burden of note creation on the software, while allowing the physician to merely make adjustments for precision. He or she can free-type additional information pertinent to the visit and can add specific symptoms or exam findings which have not been entered by default. The program can even assist in the development of a care plan, by offering decision-support and commonly prescribed medications for each assessment.

3. *Electronic dictation* – One final method worth considering – electronic dictation – has been employed by thousands of physicians with significant success. Using specialized software and a microphone, the physician can dictate directly into the EHR and the speech will be instantly converted to text. Most electronic records have built-in support for this and integrate seamlessly with the dictation software.

The most commonly used dictation product is "Dragon Naturally Speaking" by Nuance Software (www.nuance.com). While expensive, Dragon has a track record for accuracy and ease of use. For health professionals, a special medical edition has been created which includes built-in vocabulary support for all major specialties and sub-specialties. Some physicians who are already used to dictating may find this to be the perfect solution to maintain their current level of efficiency. Others may find it awkward. Unlike dictating into a small tape or a digital recorder, using software like Dragon, requires the clinician to wear a headset (either wired or wireless) for every encounter, and does take some training to build accuracy. This may create a perceived barrier to personal patient care, and raises the issue of where the dictation will take place.

In order to maintain efficiency, documentation is best done during the encounter. While this may be subtly achieved via the two afore-mentioned methods, there is nothing subtle about dictation. Some physicians may wish to avoid dictating in the exam room because it may raise questions or highlight issues that make the patient feel uncomfortable. Other providers may like the idea that the patient will know exactly what is documented to avoid any confusion over the plan of care. Consider these issues when investing in the speech recognition software, as well as how information entered by the clinical staff integrates with the dictated note. As with typing, dictation creates an end product which is very precise and readable, but may not be ideal for every office environment. These issues should be discussed and at least preliminarily decided upon before implementation, as many EHRs are built to accommodate any of the three options.

To Code or Not to Code

The method of documentation will impact billing and coding with the electronic record. Most EHRs provide suggestions to the clinician on how the visit should be charged based on current CMS guidelines. Using data entered into the note, a "level" for the visit may be offered by the software. Unfortunately, this cannot be achieved with dictated or typed notes at every instance, as programs typically rely on specific data points entered by the user to make an evaluation. In other words, the software may only know the number of historical or physical exam areas reviewed by tallying up the number of check boxes selected by the user. If the note contains only free text, this will not be possible and an accurate visit level cannot be offered.

As one of the promises of health information technology is improving charge capture and increasing revenue, it is certainly beneficial to take advantage of coding support wherever possible. Many offices may decide to delay implementing this feature at first, and continue to code manually until all users have become comfortable with the software. Either way, no EHR will completely automate the process. Input is still required by the clinician to make the final judgment on visit level, so care providers should be comfortable with how their final notes will look when generated by the program. In the end an auditor will still hold the clinician – not the software – to account for how the visit is billed.

Electronic Prescribing

One of the biggest time-savers offered by electronic records is e-prescribing. Using the EHR, a clinician can instantly renew a prescription with the click of a button. The script can then be printed out for the patient or sent electronically to the pharmacy to be filled. But, this advanced technology brings some concerns which should be addressed in the pre-implementation period to avoid serious issues later on.

First, e-prescribing may provide staff members access to a physician's electronic "prescription pad." This can be both incredibly convenient and very disturbing. To elaborate, there may be instances where a prescription needs to be corrected or simply reprinted, due to error or loss. Perhaps, the provider entered the wrong quantity for an anti-hypertensive medication, or the patient misplaced it on the way to the pharmacy. With the new technology, a staff member can correct or re-print the prescription without the need to disturb the physician. This can provide great benefit to office efficiency.

But this also opens the door for serious medical errors and even criminal activity. If a staff member does not fully understand the situation or introduces an error, there can be disastrous consequences. Improper dosages or instructions could easily be entered by even the most well-meaning individual. Even more disturbing, ill-intentioned employees could take advantage of their access for nefarious purposes, and generate their own prescriptions without consulting a physician. Even though certain medications (such as DEA schedule II narcotics) require manual signing, there are many controlled substance prescriptions which need only electronic signatures. For these reasons, practices should consider limited access to prescription generation to the clinicians and superusers. Even at the cost of efficiency, the value of ensuring a safe and secure prescribing system cannot be overstated.

Another concern worth addressing prior to implementation is the security of printed prescriptions. Unlike handwritten scripts, computer-generated prescriptions are easy to copy and forge. Even the signature may be supplied by the software, eliminating the need for the clinician to add anything to the document. If printed on plain paper, scripts can then be scanned and edited illegally by untrustworthy patients. Practices should therefore consider using special paper for printing scripts, especially those for controlled substances. Available papers should include features such as security backgrounds that display the word "void" when copied or scanned or serial numbers to track individual prescriptions. Other options to be considered include special printers which generate small documents in the size and configuration of traditional prescription pads, with the same security features mentioned above. All of these products can be pricey but can provide tremendous peace of mind and improve patient safety.

Considering a Patient Portal

Most EHR products offer the ability for patients to interact with their physician through a secure web-based portal. This may allow for scheduling appointments, requesting refills on prescriptions, or asking simple health questions. Other features include reporting lab results or following up on office visits. For example, a physician may instruct a patient to electronically submit blood glucose readings over the weeks following an office encounter. This can make communicating convenient for both the doctor and the patient, but does come with a few caveats.

First, these electronic visits (or e-visits) should not take the place of a face-to-face interaction; they should be limited to basic correspondence and information sharing. This will help prevent inappropriate messages from flooding a physician's inbox, and ensure that more complicated issues are dealt with in person. All electronic communications must pass through the portal, and personal e-mail accounts should never be used. Personal e-mail accounts are not secure and promote casual interactions, thereby jeopardizing the professional relationship between the physician and the patient.

Another issue to consider is the legal implication of communicating electronically. Unlike face-to-face or telephone conversations, e-mail correspondence lacks inflection and tone, and can be easily misconstrued if not carefully worded. It is imperative that physicians follow certain ground rules for communicating, such as those published in 2002 by the American Medical Association. Available on their website, the AMA's "Guidelines for Physician–Patient Electronic Communications" suggest that e-visits should only supplement office encounters, and that privacy issues should be discussed with patients prior to initiating electronic correspondence.

One final thought relates to how electronic visits will affect the "bottom line." Let's face it, communication takes time, and time is money. Electronic visits hopefully save time by eliminating the need for staff to field phone calls or process simple patient requests. There is also the potential for practices to be compensated for electronic encounters. Some insurers, such as Blue Cross Blue Shield of North Carolina, have recently begun reimbursing for e-visits provided certain criteria are met. Other payors, including Medicare and Medicaid, have indicated they may soon follow suit. In the mean time, physicians should be comfortable with integrating electronic encounters into their daily routine. If e-visits only lead to frustration and inefficiency, no amount of reimbursement will make them worthwhile, and the idea of implementing a patient portal should be tabled until a later time.

Preparing to "Go Paperless"

In preparation for the EHR transition, many practices are hopeful for the day when they can eliminate paper charts and truly go "paperless." Unfortunately, this can be one of the hardest steps to take in adopting this new technology, because even with the best EHR software, the process of adding old data into the system is time-consuming and far from ideal.

Consider that there are two basic methods for entering past information. Certain data such as diagnoses, medication lists, and allergies need to be manually entered by the physician or staff. Conversely, documents, such as radiology reports, correspondence, or handwritten notes must be scanned into the record. This is a labor-intensive process, and may be rife with pitfalls and stumbling blocks which should be anticipated wherever possible before getting started.

First, accept that it is impossible to transition out of paper immediately. The process of scanning old charts into the new system will be an awesome undertaking, and even if an outside company is contracted to remove this burden from the office staff, the costs may be prohibitive. To avoid an efficiency melt-down when first setting out, practices should be encouraged to "work forward" from the point of installation of the EHR. Any patient data which are acquired after the technology is implemented will avoid the paper chart altogether and be entered directly into the system. If it is discrete historical information, the physician or staff will input it manually into the appropriate location in the digital record. If it is a document or report, a staff member will immediately scan and attach it to the proper patient's electronic chart. The paper original will be destroyed instead of filing it as before. In this way, all staff will know that data obtained after the date of the EHR's installation can be found inside the computer.

Once a practice begins entering old data into the EHR, a well thought-through plan for how to proceed can pay off with significant dividends. This may include prioritizing which charts to scan first, and "prepping the charts" by filtering out irrelevant data prior to scanning. This will maximize efficiency and cost-effectiveness. For more information on creating an action plan for this process, refer to the next chapter on EHR implementation.

Final Thoughts on Pre-implementation

So far, we have considered the EHR selection and implementation process from the perspective of a solo or small-group practice. But individual offices may decide not to "go it alone." Instead, practices may join together or partner with a local health network to share bargaining power and minimize financial risk. This clearly can have advantages to smaller offices and ultimately may improve patient care.

There is no question that joining together can result in real financial benefit. EHR pricing is typically based on the number of care providers who will be using the system – the more the providers, the lower the cost per individual user – and vendors are usually willing to negotiate. More physicians mean greater leverage at the bargaining table. If the transition is spearheaded by a local health network or hospital, smaller practices can rely on the larger organization for leadership, and depend on their negotiating muscle. The hospital can also help to minimize the costs to the individual practices by providing support or data hosting services at a significantly reduced rate.

Once completed, cooperative EHR implementations can also result in greater information portability and data sharing. Consultants can easily access medications, allergies, and problems lists for individual patients without needing to contact their

PCP, while primary docs can read consultant notes as soon as they are generated. In addition, an EHR shared across a health network facilitates access to critical health data no matter where a patient seeks care. For example, an ER physician could rely on the EHR to provide essential information even when presented with an unconscious patient.

Across the country, many healthcare systems have already established Regional Health Information Organizations (RHIOs). These networks link hospitals and private practices to allow health information exchange. One large RHIO has been created in New York City and is known as The Primary Care Information Project; this ambitious undertaking has already gathered thousands of physicians under one technological umbrella. It allows primary docs and specialists to access patient information and communicate electronically, and even permits patients to review and update their personal records through an online portal. In the long run, doctors expect the project to deliver better outcomes and higher quality care.

To Sum Up...

This chapter underscores the premise that preparation is the key to success. In the world of HIT, this notion is critical. Avoiding failure when implementing an EHR is dependent on asking the right questions long before taking the first step and continually re-evaluating the answers to those questions along the way. With a focus on teamwork, and a healthy amount of enthusiasm, practices can create buy-in and ownership of the process and ensure employee satisfaction. Ultimately, it is not the limitations of technology that leads to the untimely demise of EHR installations. Instead, failure is caused by impaired office efficiency, frustrated staff, and decreased physician satisfaction resulting from not taking the proper steps to prepare along the way.

Chapter 5
Implementation

Anupam Kashyap

> There is certain relief in change, even though it be from bad to
> worse! As I have often found in traveling in a stagecoach, that it
> is often a comfort to shift one's position, and be bruised in a
> new place.
> — Washington Irving, Tales of a Traveler (1824)

Abstract Implementing an EMR is probably the most difficult, significant, and potentially beneficial change a practice can make. The change has wide-ranging impact on the experience of everyone in the office, from physicians to staff, and to patients. When done correctly it can yield benefits on the quality of patient care, ease of charting, and improvement in revenue. When done wrong, it creates longer working hours, decreased revenue, across the board employee dissatisfaction with work, and encroachment upon the personal time. Making any change to a large extent is never easy, and most physicians describe starting an EMR in their practice as one of the most difficult organizational experiences that their practice had to face. This chapter will emphasize the practical tools and tips for implementing an EMR to increase your chances of success and minimize the pain. The recommendations in this chapter are drawn from the lessons we have learnt in implementing EMRs for over 30,000 physicians over the last 10 years. There is no need to reinvent the wheel. There are proven methodologies of doing it right. In this section, we will discuss how to assess the symptoms or aspects of a practice that need attention during a successful implementation, examine how to develop and deliver a treatment plan for those aspects of practice that is not limited to the first day of implementation but one that provides continuity of care to the health of your office in becoming proficient and maximizing the utilization of tools an EMR provides.

Keywords EMR implementation · Physician and staff buy-in · Meaningful use criteria · Chart preparation

A. Kashyap (✉)
Director of Implementation eClinicalWorks, 140 Broadway, New York, NY 10005, USA
e-mail: anupam@eclinicalworks.com

N.S. Skolnik (ed.), *Electronic Medical Records*, Current Clinical Practice,
DOI 10.1007/978-1-60761-606-1_5, © Springer Science+Business Media, LLC 2011

Implementing an EMR is probably the most difficult, significant, and potentially beneficial change a practice can make. The change has wide ranging impact on the experience of everyone in the office, from physicians to staff, and to patients. When done correctly it can yield benefits on the quality of patient care, ease of charting, and improvement in revenue. When done wrong, it creates longer working hours, decreased revenue, and across the board employee dissatisfaction with work, and encroachment upon the personal time. Making any change to a large extent is never easy, and most physicians describe starting an EMR in their practice as one of the most difficult organizational experiences that their practice had to face. Implementing an EMR requires a lot of patience and acceptance of short-term inconveniences and pain, in order to get through the initial implementation stage. Knowing this ahead of time allows you to prepare the office for such short-term pain with a vision of long-term gain. Everyone, in every position in the office, must be convinced of the benefits of EMR to patient care, and to their own position in the office in order to sustain the dedication necessary to get through the transition phase which inevitably will involve a few weekends and late nights preparing for EMR adoption, and will often test your patience when things don't go right. Transformational change of this type requires careful planning and preparation for both the predictable and the unpredictable experiences of stress.

It is very possible that during first few days of implementation, many in the office will consider or suggest quitting the process and going back to the comfort zone of paper charting. At these times, the physician leader needs to remind himself or herself, as well as others about the core reasons why the practice decided for transition to an EMR in the first place and the potential benefits for the practice and for patients.

This chapter will emphasize the practical tools and tips for implementing an EMR to increase your chances of success and minimize the pain. The recommendations in this chapter are drawn from the lessons we have learnt in implementing EMRs for over 30,000 physicians over the last 10 years. There is no need to re-invent the wheel. There are proven methodologies of doing it right. In this section, we will discuss how to assess the symptoms or aspects of a practice that need attention during a successful implementation, examine how to develop, and deliver a treatment plan for those aspects of practice that is not limited to the first day of implementation but one that provides continuity of care to the health of your office in becoming proficient and maximizing the utilization of tools an EMR provides.

It is important to have clear short- and long-term goals. The short-term goal is the successful adoption of an EMR with the smallest amount and shortest period of pain and practice disruption possible. The long-term goal is to be a meaningful user of EMR. The difference is using the system versus using the system well to deliver desirable patient care outcomes.

Becoming a meaningful user of EMR is no different from treating a patient and managing his/her health over a period of time. You have to listen carefully and gather the characteristics of a successful implementation, review the systems that are critical to success, make assessment of the problems you might face, define a treatment plan for each system reviewed, act upon them, and then measure and improve.

Let's first identify the symptoms or characteristics of a successful implementation and then we will address each one in more detail. The most important one is the buy-in from the physicians and staff members. Without a firm sense of buy-in, it is unlikely that physician and staff morale will remain at a reasonable level during the arduous process of implementation. How committed are the physicians and staff members? How much should you involve them in the process?

The second important aspect of implementation is adjusting patient schedules. There are several questions you need to ask yourself; do I need to cut down my patient load? When? How much and for how long? Is there any creative way to minimize financial impact of not seeing enough patients and yet be able to focus on learning and adjusting to new workflows revolving around this new electronic system?

The third aspect is chart preparation. Should the practice start with a clean slate on day one in EMR? Or should some patient data be pre-loaded ahead of time? Is it good enough to scan patient charts? Or should we consider entering discrete data in the EMR? What's the best strategy to prepare charts for EMR to go live?

The fourth one is commitment to training. Is it worthwhile not to see patients and be trained on EMR? How much time should be spent in classroom training? How much time should be spent on hands-on training? Is there anything that can be done to minimize the reduction of patient visits during training? What is the best strategy to get trained on an EMR?

The fifth one is the value of a super-user. How would it help to have super-users? How many are needed? And what should be done to develop super-users?

Let us now address each one of these important issues in turn.

1. Physician and staff buy-in:

EMRs are merely tools without people and process. It is the people that make it work. It is most critical that everyone involved is bought into it and that there is some level of involvement. There needs to be a sense of ownership by the users and the users need to share the drive to make it work. You should work with your vendor to conduct system demonstrations and provide everyone an opportunity to get familiar, ask questions, and mentally start preparing for having the system in place. You do not want to stop the communication there. Involve your staff in the workflow assessment and re-design process. Involve them in developing patient communication about the EMR adoption. Often vendors have online sessions for basic of using the system. Plan to have your staff to attend these sessions. Work with your vendor to provide a "play environment" for users to log in at their convenience and play with the system. Playing with the system ahead of time allows them to learn the system before there is the added pressure of patients waiting while the system is being negotiated for the first time. Develop momentum and keep the momentum going as the project unfolds and moves toward the start date. Keep all physicians and staff informed on the progress of the project so that everyone feels that they have an important stake in the process. Continue to remind people of the original vision for the EMR, of the benefits so that the ultimate goals of implementing an EMR are truly integrated with the goals of the practice and are goals that all members of the physician and office staff fully understand, and remain in the forefront of everyone's minds.

2. Adjustments in patient schedule:
Cutting down patient schedules impact the following systems:

- *Revenue*: In an ideal world, you don't want any negative impact on revenue at all. Therefore, your tendency would be not to reduce patient schedule or to the least possible amount. Unfortunately, it is almost impossible to have a successful implementation without some disruption in schedules.
- *Ability to learn the system and adjust to new workflows*: During go-live you are still learning the system and the whole new workflows. You are still getting used to the new way of interacting with the patient, staff, other physicians, and technology. This part wants the freedom to adapt and learn and not be pressured by the pace of patients flowing into your examination room, while you are still figuring out what your trainer taught you and where to find the medication you'd like to prescribe or the diagnosis that you can't seem to find.
- *Medical errors as a result of not knowing the system well*: One of the most frightening possibilities with a new system is that of making a medical error because of poor knowledge of how the system works. This possibility is one of the strongest arguments for intelligently adjusting the patient schedule when starting a new EMR so as to allow for the time it takes to simply "find" the test or medication in a system that is new to you. The worst scenario is feeling behind and rushed and now knowing how to order a test or prescribe a medication effectively. Anticipating this is important in order to allow time in the schedule to accommodate for this.
- *Managing the stress of completing notes and seeing all scheduled patients in a timely fashion*: You can get overwhelmed by the amount of patients you have to see and notes that are needed to document the visits, electronic prescriptions that need to be written, lab or radiology orders, referrals, and tracking down and viewing past results in a new system where each click and task involved figures out something new. It is not unusual for patient visits to take longer, and by the afternoon you can even become more behind and backed up than usual.
- *Patients who are sick still need medical help*: All said and done; patients who need urgent care or walk in, still need to be seen and provided medical care.

There are inherent conflicts in the choices one must make around these issues. Minimizing the impact on revenue will maximize the opportunity for stress, frustration, and medical errors, while decreasing the opportunity to become comfortable with the EMR and have patients participate with some satisfaction with the visit and the introduction of the EMR into the office. After examining the above-defined systems and the office one must define a plan that strikes a balance between conflicting priorities.

A plan that often works in striking the right balance between maximizing the opportunity to learn and getting going as soon as possible to the point where you start reaping the benefits of an EMR is shown in Table 5.1.

Table 5.1 Patient scheduling plan

Go-live patient scheduling plan		Week 1	Week 2	Week 3	Week 4	Week 5
Patient schedule adjustment		50%	60%	70%	80%	100%
Patient visit duration adjustment	15-min visit	30 min	25 min	20 min	20 min	15 min
	30-min visit	60 min	50 min	45 min	40 min	30 min
	45-min visit	90 min	75 min	65 min	55 min	45 min

Start with a 50% patient load in the first week of your EMR adoption. Increase it by 10% every week and bring up the patient load back to original by fifth week of using the EMR. This is a guideline that should be adjusted based on computer proficiency of users, ability to learn and adjust, the EMR you select, and the workflow integrations and chart preparation done prior to go-live, which will be discussed in more detail later.

Sometimes the cost of cutting down patient visits can add up to thousands of dollars, depending on your patient mix and reimbursement rates. As you anticipate the real costs of EMR implementation, it is also important to take these costs into account. We will use some assumptions and to show how to calculate the revenue hit in order to anticipate what to account for in your budget. Let's assume that each provider sees 30 patients in a day, 13 of which are 15-min visits at Medicare reimbursement of $48 per visit, 10 of which are 30-min visits at Medicare reimbursement of $55 per visit, 7 of which are 45-min visits at Medicare reimbursement of $60 per visit. Table 5.2 is a guide for calculation.

In this example, before going live if you were seeing 13 patients for 15 min follow-up visits and getting reimbursed $48 per visit, your week 1 patient load would be seven follow-up visits, going up to eight in week 2, 10 in weeks 3 and 4, and back to 13 in week 5. Note that this is an example to help you plan ahead. You certainly don't want to be in cash crunch in the middle of your EMR go-live. The solution is either to budget for it ahead of time or be creative and use your friends and colleague physicians who have recently gone live on the same system or in the process to provide extra coverage during the go-live at your practice.

3. Chart preparation:
Preparing charts for the EMR involves data abstraction from paper charts and entering clinical information important to treating the patient into the electronic chart. Preparing charts for patient visits in an EMR has great advantage and is highly recommended, but it costs time and therefore money. The systems that influence the decisions are

- *Duration of patient visit*: If you decide not to prepare charts for EMR go-live, your patient visits will be longer than if you transfer information to the chart

Table 5.2 Projected revenue impact of EMR implementation

Impact on revenue	Number of visits/day	Reimbursement/ visit	Week 1		Week 2		Week 3		Week 4	
			Number of visits/day	Weekly drop in revenue	Number of visits/day	Weekly drop in revenue	No. visits/day	Weekly drop in revenue	No. visits/day	Weekly drop in revenue
15-min visit	13	$48	7	$1,440	8	$1,248	10	$780	10	$780
30-min visit	10	$55	5	$1,375	6	$1,100	7	$917	8	$688
45-min visit	7	$60	4	$900	4	$840	5	$646	6	$382
Total impact per provider				$11,095						

ahead of time. Recognize that longer patient visits result in lower productivity, greater impact on revenue, and also impact patient satisfaction.

- *Resource cost for preparing charts*: If you do prepare charts, you end-up spending your personal time in office for 4–6 weeks or pay staff to scan and pre-load data into the EMR.
- *Pre-load versus scanning*: While scanning is easy, pre-loading patient data into the correct fields will result in building patient medical records that are easy to update, and also facilitate reports and decision-support systems. The other thing to consider is how easy it is to get to a scanned chart and flip through the scanned chart electronically.
- *Reliability of data pre-loaded*: Whom do you trust most to pre-load the clinical data? Is it your nurse, medical assistant, clerk, or a medical student you know? Or you trust nobody but yourself? This is an issue that needs to be discussed carefully among the physicians prior to implementation and the answer to this question is different for every office and is influenced by the resources available and the comfort of the physicians with letting clinical information being entered into the medical record by someone other than a physician. If non-physician staff are given the responsibility to enter data, that clinical data must be reviewed by the physicians at some point, since the physician is ultimately responsible for the integrity of the information in the medical record.

It is clear that the value of preparing the chart overshadows the cost. The question is not whether to prepare but rather how to prepare. The questions revolve around finding the right balance for your practice between the cost of transferring pre-existing paper-based information to the EMR prior to go-live and what can be done as you are live and going along seeing patients. What follows is a recommended approach which should be adapted to individual practice needs.

Start with a spreadsheet and list down the critical components of your chart. Below is an example of how your list should look like and my recommendations for when to consider transferring medicine to the electronic system (Table 5.3).

For scanning documents from patient chart, consider the following process: Identify the charts that have components that need to be scanned by affixing a sticker. Use stickers to identify which documents in the chart should be scanned into the EMR. Make sure all staff members involved in scanning are familiar with a standard nomenclature that is to be used for all scanned documents. You do not want one person scanning a chest X-ray from April 7, 2008 with a file name of "Chest X-ray April 2008" while another staff member might file it as "X-ray, Chest 2007 Apr". One solution that many practice use is naming scanned documents by date (mm/dd/year, category, sub-category). For example

02/03/2008 Radiology Chest
02/22/2008 Consults Pulmonary
03/23/2008 Radiology CAT Scan Chest

Table 5.3 Sample spreadsheet for transferring medical charts into an electronic system

Define what's important to bring forward from patient record. Define what to scan, what to import electronically, what can be entered as data. Define the resource to perform the function.						
Chart preparation items	Ability of EMR to store discrete data	Recommended method to use	For which patients?	Recommended resource	When to start?	Comments
Problem list	Yes	Data entry	Patients scheduled for next three months and patients with chronic conditions like diabetes, hypertension	Clinical staff enters and provider reviews	Entry: 4–6 weeks prior to visit. Review: During patient's first visit	If reliable clinical resources do not exist then clinicians should enter information themselves
	No	Scan	All	Medical records staff	4–6 weeks prior to patient visit	
Rx history	Yes	Import	All	Provider	At the time of first visit	Some EMRs have ability to import medication history. If your EMR doesn't, the next best option is to allow medical staff to enter it a day before the patient visit and you review and update it during patient visit
	No	Scan	Patients scheduled for next three months and patients with chronic conditions like diabetes, hypertension	Medical records staff	4–6 weeks prior to patient visit	
Immunization/vaccination history	Yes	Data entry/import	ALL	Nurse	4–6 weeks prior to patient visit	Optionally you can work with your City Immunization Registry to get data you have been reporting to them and vendor to import it. You can review and update during patient visit
	No	Scan	ALL	Medical records staff	4–6 weeks prior to patient visit	
Allergies	Yes	Data Entry	ALL	MA	At the time of first visit	
	No	Scan	ALL	Medical records staff	4–6 weeks prior to patient visit	

Table 5.3 (continued)

	Yes	Bubble sheet/data entry	ALL	MA	At the time of first visit	Some EMRs have ability to import histories using bubble sheets
Medical history						
	No	Scan	ALL	Medical records staff	4–6 weeks prior to patient visit	
Hospitalization history	Yes	Bubble sheet/data entry	ALL	MA	At the time of first visit	Some EMRs have ability to import histories using bubble sheets
	No	Scan	ALL	Medical records staff	4–6 weeks prior to patient visit	
	Yes	Bubble sheet/data entry	ALL	MA	At the time of first visit	Some EMRs have ability to import histories using bubble sheets
Family history						
	No	Scan	ALL	Medical records staff	4–6 weeks prior to patient visit	
	Yes	Bubble sheet/data entry	ALL	MA	At the time of first visit	Some EMRs have ability to import histories using bubble sheets
Surgical history						
	No	Scan	ALL	Medical records staff	4–6 weeks prior to patient visit	
Charts/progress notes	N/A	Scan	None	None		Alternatively you scan last three progress notes. Also, it is recommended that you keep paper charts (for reference only) for six months to a year. This will act as your safety net and at the same time minimizes what you have to scan and just be able to refer to it at the point of care
Last colonoscopy/mammogram/EKG	Yes	Data entry	As needed	Providers/MA		Enter it as part of training or can be done as you see patient
	No	Data entry	As needed	Medical records staff	4–6 weeks prior to patient visit	

Whatever system of naming is chosen, it is imperative that everyone in the practice know the system and abides by it in order to be able to easily file and find material that is scanned.

Once a chart has had its necessary contents scanned into the EMR, not further incoming paper should be put in the chart, as the incoming paper should go directly into the EMR.

After a chart has been scanned, it is still a good idea to have access to the paper chart as a backup to look for information for up to a year. The chart should be used though strictly for reference and not new information should be added to the paper chart.

Most of the practices and provider's who have done well in adopting EMRs have made intelligent use of both paper and electronic worlds during preparation, training, and adoption.

4. Onsite training:

Commitment to training: If you want to reap the maximal benefits of the money and effort that have been put into selecting and purchasing an EMR, you have to acknowledge that you will have to spend a lot of time learning how to use the system. Since this is going to change the way that you practice medicine more than any other single thing that you have encountered since you went to medical school, you will have to acknowledge that you will have to spend a lot of time and effort to make the EMR work. Commit to spending a period of concentrated time focusing on learning. When the trainer from the vendor is in your office, free yourself up and make use of that valuable time-limited opportunity. Try not to dilute the time by scheduling patient visits to conflict with the time you have put aside to lean the system, no matter how tempting it would seem to do that. Everyone has a different way of learning, so try to adapt this experience to work best with the personal styles of the physicians and staff in your office. Some people have graphic memories, not needing to make notes, but remembering what it is that they saw someone do. Others learn best by reading, others by having things explained, and still others only by hands-on experience. Whatever is your style of learning, make sure you discuss it with your trainer. Usually, trainers are very patient and have experience with adapting their style based on the learning style of trainees. Remember that the trainer is there to facilitate your learning their EMR. You need to make yourself and your staff available and if any particular styles of leaning the system seem like it would work best for you, let the trainer know.

Big bang roll-out versus phased roll-out: You have a choice to train everyone on the complete system and get everyone live at the same time, or break the training into pieces and the go-live into logical phases. If your EMR is also your registration, scheduling, and billing system, it might make sense to start with the non-clinical portion of training and get the front office, medical records, office manager, billing staff trained and start using the system. The EMR portion of the system can then be started the next week or after 2–4 weeks, depending on the costs involved and EMR vendor recommendations.

If you take the phased approach, which often works well, you can use that opportunity to continue to improve your skills with the EMR by using some portion of EMR while operational staff is going live. Parts to start with might be e-prescription, messaging, charge capture, and reviewing electronic lab results.

Phased approach allows you and your staff to learn and adopt small increments of the system and results in better change management. If you have multiple locations, one consideration is to keep a 2-week gap between implementation at different locations and use the opportunity to capture and communicate the lessons learned at one location to the subsequent locations.

For training, follow the five-point plan below:

- *Follow a set agenda*: Define a set agenda for training, working with your project manager and trainer. Identify the training requirements and best practices. Identify the roles your staff play in your office and structure the training by their roles. Ensure that your trainer is well versed with your workflows, before starting the training. Make sure that your EMR trainer from your EMR vendor has spent time in your office, so he or she understands your current workflow and can help you to adapt the EMR to your office work patterns and your current work patterns to work better with the EMR. While there is no single best workflow process, you can be certain that many of your current processes will have to change to adapt to the needs of your new EMR system. Organize your training based on workflows in the office instead of learning different modules of the system. Provide your trainer with some typical scenarios and workflows. The training time will vary depending on the EMR system you get. Expect to spend at least 8–12 h in physician training. Expect your staff to be in training for similar amount of time. Plan the training well enough in advance so that you can re-schedule your patients or make alternative arrangements for your patients, during your training days. Communicate to your staff when they are scheduled for training. Also, clarify a go-live date for the EMR. Define go-live clearly to your staff. If you work with your medical assistant or nurse as a team and rely a lot on her/him, plan on including your assistant in physician training sessions.
- *Meaningful use criteria*: Work with your EMR project manager and trainer to incorporate training on modules that empower you to meet meaningful use definition. Ideally the workflows and training scenarios should be prepared ahead of time to include the key features and modules that count toward meaningful use of an EMR. Create a checklist to verify that you and your staff got trained appropriately. Different vendors have different degrees of meticulousness with regard to training so to the degree that you can define, and have a checklist of the areas that you want to make sure to know about to have a better chance of having all those areas covered.
- *Clear yours and staff's schedule*: Make sure you clear your schedule completely and no patients are scheduled during training. There is nothing worse than having to walk out during an important part of a training session and then having everyone in the room suffer having to go over that material again when you walk back in. If you are a solo-physician office, you might feel that there is no way you can shut down your entire office and loose revenue for a training session. The problem is there is not much choice if you intend to learn the EMR system quickly and get back to your usual level of efficiency in seeing patients in an electronic world. As difficult as it is, the truth is that the sooner and more efficiently you learn how to work in your known system, the soon it will be that you will be able to obtain the benefits of the EMR that lead you to decide to get an EMR in the first place. If needed, arrange coverage. If you have two or more physicians in

your office, you can divide the office into more than one team. While one team is in training, the other one attends to patients. In this way you can balance training and running the office. Regardless of what your situation is, it is absolutely important that you are not in and out of training. Clear your schedule and commit yourself to learning.

- *Secure a training space*: You will need a space which will provide you and your staff the ability to focus on learning, without distraction; ability to have your training workstations or laptops or tablet PC; and any other training equipment like scanners/printers/projector that your trainer needs in the room. Understand the training requirements ahead of time and secure a training space accordingly. Regardless of what EMR you get, keep the training groups small, allowing the trainer to provide optimal attention to each individual.

- *Motivate your staff*: Moving your entire operations from a paper world to an electronic world is a monumental task. Change doesn't come easy, and remember that both physicians and staff would need on-going support and re-motivation. Some might just need a little encouragement, some might need pizza or donuts and coffee, and some may even need a shoulder to cry. The point is to identify what motivates your staff and have a plan in place to keep everyone together in learning and adopting a new world of EMR with a sense that you are moving together into the future of medicine.

- *Leverage your super-users*: Early in your implementation, identify users who have interests in certain functions which they are likely to learn and adopt quicker than others. Give them a head start in learning the system. Check with your project manager to see if any online tools like webinars, videos, or documentation are available for training for those in your staff who are self-motivated and want to do more. Check to see if as a part of the training the project manager or trainer can provide early or additional training for your super-users. During training and go-live, super-users provide an important source of extra assistance to the staff and can serve as a funnel point for questions from staff to the EMR vendor.

- *Conduct surveys*: Surveys before and after training will provide you insight into what's working and what's not. Survey your patients, physician, and staff on their experience.

- *Reduce patient load*: It's not only useful to reduce patient load during training, but also for several weeks into go-live, as we addressed earlier in the chapter. There is a learning curve to any new system. You won't be proficient immediately after training to go back to full patient load. The time it takes for a physician to get back to full load of patients varies from one EMR to another. Our suggestions have been to decrease patient appointments by 50% in week 1 of go-live, and increase it by 10–15% every week, based on your assessment of how well the adoption is. It will take you at least 4–5 weeks to get back to normal.

- *Manage patient expectations*: Inform your patients in advance that you are adopting an EMR. Educate them on the benefits like e-prescription, electronic lab orders and results, improved communication with them, reduced paperwork and waiting time, etc. Alert them that during go-live weeks, there could be potential delays as everyone gets familiar with the new system. Ask them to be patient. Post some flyers in waiting areas. For most part, the patients are usually supportive and excited to see their practice entering the computer age. It's important to include patient communication part of your implementation strategy. It is also not a bad idea to suggest to patients to double-check their prescriptions during the first few months after the system goes live, as the potential for medications errors increases during the time period where information is being transferred from paper charts to electronic charts and a new way of writing prescriptions is being learned. It is also reasonable to re-assure patients that ultimately electronic prescribing is less prone to error and is safer than paper-based prescribing, but that early on in the new system it is simply a good idea for everyone to be extra cautious.

- *Importance of electronic lab results*: Plan EMR go-live along with lab integration with EMR. CPOE is one of the key components of the meaningful use definition. Getting results on paper once you are using EMR makes you and your staff's life much harder to manage with additional scanning and data entry of results. Pay attention to progress of lab integration right through the implementation. This also helps you in utilizing preventive service alerts in the system, at the point of patient care, if the EMR has one.

5. Availability of "super-users":

One of the factors that distinguish a successful implementation from more difficult ones is the interest and availability of super-users. Super-users are those members of the practice who have taken the initiative to receive further training in the use of the EMR and serve as a resource for others in the practice. Developing super-users for different functional areas will benefit the practice, make implementation easier, provide an ongoing resource for the practice, and is often a source of significant job satisfaction for the individuals identified as super-users who are now able to further help their colleges in important ways. The easiest way to identify super-users is to ask staff about their interest in becoming a super-user and their experience with computers. Usually the two go hand in hand. The second characteristic of a super-user is their willingness to help. Third one is their interest in actively participating in improving various aspects of EMR adoption by staff. As long as someone who is interested seems to have reasonable computer experience, and is well respected in the office, it is a good idea to utilize their interests and help them in developing their skills as a super-user.

Get the super-users trained as early as 4 weeks into the implementation. Make sure they have access to a sandbox or play environment of the system immediately after their training. This is to ensure that the learning doesn't fade away with time.

Utilize super-users in (a) workflow analysis, (b) training preparation, (c) system build, (d) training, go-live and ongoing in-house support to staff members, and (e) ongoing changes in system customizations.

We discussed the importance of workflow analysis, re-design and training based on workflows, in previous chapters. You can potentially utilize your super-users to help you with each of these processes. Super-users can assist in adapting the EMR based on the gaps identified in the workflow analysis and re-design process. Super-users can also work on creating spreadsheets for training and go-live. When the EMR trainers are gone, the super-users will act as the safety net for your staff as they get comfortable with the system and new workflow.

Before we move into the "Maintenance and Optimization" chapter, it is important to understand that success with implementation is an outcome of the practices approach and does not reflect the efforts of any one person alone. Difficult choices have to be made as a group. If answers to these questions exist they lie in compromise among the members of the group, and in ongoing discussions that find a balance between cost and value. This chapter should have provided important tools and tricks to address some of the most critical and challenging aspects of an EMR implementation. Prepared for the difficulty of the journey, the journey sometimes is not as difficult as it might otherwise have been.

Chapter 6
Maintenance and Optimization

Thomas M. Wilkinson

*The greatest danger in times of turbulence is not the turbulence;
it is to act with yesterday's logic.*
– Peter Drucker, management consultant and writer

Abstract This chapter is the "owner's manual" part of this book. You might study the physics of dynamic equilibrium, but that does not teach you how to ride a bike. So after months or even years of study and planning, you might know plenty about EMRs, but until you are in the driver's seat, you really will not know much about how to use them. You will need to know which circumstances are good to use them, which are not, how they function, what the rules of the road are, how to take care of them, and even how to make them better.

Keywords EMR maintenance · EMR optimization · Physician champion · Super user · EMR management

Introduction

This chapter is the "owner's manual" part of this book. You might study the physics of dynamic equilibrium, but that does not teach you how to ride a bike. So after months or even years of study and planning, you might know plenty about EMRs, but until you are in the driver's seat, you really will not know much about how to use them. You will need to know which circumstances are good to use them, which are not, how they function, what the rules of the road are, how to take care of them, and even how to make them better.

T.M. Wilkinson (✉)
St. Mary's Hospital, 25500 Point Lookout Rd., Leonardtown, MD 20650, USA
e-mail: tmwilkinson@pol.net

N.S. Skolnik (ed.), *Electronic Medical Records*, Current Clinical Practice,
DOI 10.1007/978-1-60761-606-1_6, © Springer Science+Business Media, LLC 2011

There are probably a hundred websites to help you buy an EMR for every single website to help you actually use one. Ask a question regarding the continuous improvement of your EMR and you will hear the crickets chirping. Maintenance and optimization are virtually neglected by vendors and IT consultants, despite this phase being perhaps the most essential for ultimate success. The omission reflects an implicit assumption that after you implement an EMR and navigate the learning curve, you are somehow catapulted into a "happily-ever-after" stasis.

That is a fairy tale. Instead you enter a dynamic, iterative (and probably interminable) phase of adjustments, trials, feedback, and re-adjustments. And we do not have a national infrastructure to support you yet, and we are at best only on the verge of the transformation of EMRs from a novelty to a truly useful tool. Features become obsolete quickly, and our culture has not enveloped and incorporated the technology yet. Meanwhile, while all those aspects are maturing, there is considerable danger of injuring patients, a transformational hazard that is unique to our industry.

This chapter of the book has some areas of overlap from previous chapters, because the planning phases discussed in the beginning of this book are recapitulated in how you use the technology here. In many ways, reading this chapter first – knowing your destination – might better inform your decisions during those earlier planning phases, especially with regard to how much this is really going to cost you. The sad truth is, as much work as it took to get you here, the real work actually begins now.

The DesRoches data (see Chapter 1) showed that as of 2008, only 4% of ambulatory physicians were using a full EMR, with only an additional 13% using a partial system. Once adopted, EMRs also have high catastrophic failure rates, meaning the software is too often simply abandoned. The conservative estimates are nearly one in five, and some estimates place the failure rate between 30 and 50%. If there is any good news, this is down from the 75% failure rate from 2003. Most failures are due to a lack of successfully blending the technology with workflow; however, patient care failures (worsening outcomes) can also occur. The maintenance and optimization phase of your EMR implementation is a resource-intense requirement, and cannot be overlooked if you wish to avoid becoming part of the failure statistics.

This chapter is divided into the three short sections. The first establishes the mindset necessary to approach your EMR and use it daily. This might seem more theoretical than practical, but understanding the EMR will help moderate your frustrations, and it can potentially liberate your use of the EMR to becoming a unique blend of technology and methods, adapted to your actual needs, rather than to what the vendor has envisioned for you. The second section fleshes out details of maintenance, emphasizing the many facets of governance and management. The third section is about optimization and continuous improvement. Here is where the reasons you bought an EMR are finally realized, and I review what is necessary to secure clinical and financial outcomes.

Truly practical advice in this chapter would require knowing exactly which EMR you implemented and what your particular circumstances are. This chapter is therefore practical only inasmuch as it provides a guiding framework and might point out things that you have not already considered. There is one overarching impera- tive however, and that is to document everything you do. I recognize that you might have thought you were abandoning paper, but as you will see below, that is not realistically going to happen. Meanwhile your documentation becomes your lifeline against down-time, vendor disruptions, or EMR failures, and best captures the part of this process that belongs to you alone.

Mindset

OK, you have plugged it in and turned it on. Let's take 'er for a spin. Your partner was on call last night, so you are fully rested, you have arrived early, and you have your cup of joe. The vendor suggested booking half hour appointments for your entire first day, so you have only got 15 on the schedule – a walk in the park. You are just considering how this is going to be a triumphant day when all hell breaks loose.

Your first patient is an adult asthma exacerbation. The patient was instructed to walk in before office hours by your on-call partner, who is not awake yet to explain herself. Your front desk is in an uproar, because the patient was not pre-loaded into the system for today, and since the patient can barely speak for himself, they are scrambling to find his old paper chart. Meanwhile you interview the patient between wheezes, try to find evidence of actual air in the lungs on exam, and get a neb started. Shortly thereafter you realize that you have already missed your first opportunity to document at the point of care. The front desk now has the patient in the system, but for the life of them cannot figure out how to get him on the schedule. The scheduling templates will not let them book someone before office hours, and they cannot remember how to double book the first appointment.

Finally, 45 minutes later, the patient is breathing(!) and the EMR is finally ready(!!). So you catch up on the documentation and try to prescribe a steroid taper. Now you are really stuck. There is no obvious way to do it, so you put in a call to your technical support, but they are not up yet, since they are on California time. Your partner finally arrives and complains loudly that there is no place for her to document her on-call interaction with this patient, but she does help you with work- ing out the steroid taper – make each step a different prescription. Great idea, until every single step fires a new drug duplication alert, and 12 minutes later, the EMR wants you to print five pages for the prescription. Mental note: create a steroid taper order set. Unwilling to kill the trees, you go to the file cabinet and retrieve a single sheet copy of your well-used pre-printed taper prescription, fill it out and hand it to the patient in under 12 seconds. That took exactly one-sixtieth as much time.

Well, now you are 30 minutes behind, but you can explain it as an aberration to your usual flow. The next patient is bread-and-butter: a COPD vasculopath with high cholesterol, hypertension, CHF, and Stage II kidney disease. During the planning phase you even built templates for a few of these diagnoses, but then your excitement wanes when you cannot figure out which one to start with, or how to blend them all together. Mental note: the CHF template needs to better accommodate diminished renal function. You struggle on through, getting still further behind.

By the end of the day, you have made the following discoveries: (1) You cannot prescribe compounded meds like Magic Mouthwash. (2) Bactrim suspension, common as it seems to you, isn't on the formulary. (3) It takes an Act of Congress (or more precisely, the vendor has to "unlock" a patient record) to transfer information accidentally entered in the wrong chart back into the right one. If only you had not been interrupted by that phone call about a different patient in the first place... (4) You cannot sketch on the EKG to point out where the new changes are. (5) There are about a zillion common diagnoses which you cannot find using your usual nomenclature while searching the EMR's ICD list. I guess that is why there are professional coders, but it sure is slowing down the EMR's "bill on the fly" feature. (6) Your helpful medical assistant made up a diagnosis just to get the ABN to print, so he could vaccinate a Medicare patient. Another Act of Congress... (7) There is no way to add insulin pump or CPAP settings to the meds list. (8) A mouse is a horrible tool to try to sketch cellulitis with. (9) The automated features of the EMR turned your simple pre-op H&P into seven pages of nonsense. (10) Abilify is listed as aripiprazole, which you mistook for one of the new PPIs. Great. One last Act of Congress before going home tonight.

You only saw 12 patients, but you feel like it was 40. Your partner wants to quit. Your senior secretary hates you, since she had to reschedule three patients for you in the midst of all the chaos. Your MA wants to cry, in a manly way. Your head is pounding, your inbox is already stuffed with what amounts to EMR spam, and your morning coffee is still sitting exactly where you left it, stone cold. You are ready to pull the plug. And you had *prepared* for this day. Was it just you? Or maybe it was just the patients were peculiar today?

It turns out that every day is an aberrant day in primary care. Or, to spin it the other way, your EMR might work well for an average, idealized patient encounter, but it does not work well for the patients you actually have. Your office is a finely evolved ecosystem for health care delivery, and the EMR is an asteroid impact. It is not just a matter of reengineering your processes, although that can mitigate the shock; EMRs are simply not designed to think like you, and it gives you a huge advantage to recognize that fact up front. So, it is not you after all.

There are only one solution here that does not involve incendiary devices. Be patient. Learn. Understand the EMR and your workload. Do not try to jump from horses at the smithy's shop to the minivan at the mall without first going through buckets of gasoline and the Model T. This is going to take a sociotechnical evolution.

So let us start at the beginning. The medical record originally arose from the lab scientist's notebook. Its purpose was to record and reflect upon observations. It was, and is still supposed to be, a forum for medical reasoning. Why else would browsing the chart help us before we walk into an examination room?

EMRs do not encourage browsing, or much medical reasoning at all, for that matter. Most represent a black hole for information: they consume all data within reach of their event horizons, but no intelligible information ever seems to come back out. Actionable knowledge is certainly not a "byproduct" of using these systems, no matter what the IT lobby may have testified to Congress. EMRs are much better at documenting the Greenwich Mean Time of when a temperature was taken than they are at informing you that the patient has a fever. Simply put, EMRs are not built to support how we think, and sadly, it is our own doing.

We are suffering from a schizophrenia over our fidelity to science and our care for the specific patient sitting before us. We proclaim ourselves to be disciples of evidence-based medicine, but every practicing physician recognizes at some level that unique patients require unique solutions. We do not straight-jacket our patients into the evidence. Instead, we reconcile the science of molecular interactions with their chaotic fizz, and the science of statistical abstractions with their generalizations with the humanly scaled and very distinctive needs of our patients. And this reconciliation requires interpretive judgment as much as raw data, perhaps even more so, but we forgot to mention that.

EMRs embody the underlying assumptions of system designers, medical knowledge theorists, and administrators about how we practice, most of it marching to our incessant EBM drumming. EMRs are designed for data-driven, sequential, linear, and to put it bluntly, *rational*, thinking. Unfortunately, this conflicts with the actual nature of our work. The provision of healthcare to a patient is fundamentally gist-driven, interrupted, opportunistic, diffuse, and bluntly, *subjective*, thinking. It is nearly impossible for an EMR to help make real decisions about real patients, and yet here we are.

There are now nearly 20 years of research into medical decision making and expert reasoning consolidated under the rubric of the Fuzzy Trace Theory. These studies have shown that physicians routinely rely upon hierarchies of the *meaning* of information, "gist reasoning," rather than the verbatim details, when making clinical decisions. Moreover, there is clear evidence that excessive reliance on verbatim memory can actually impair reasoning ability, and EMRs are verbatim machines.

Let me anchor it with a simple example. An EMR approaches a patient as if she were a project to be managed. One tool commonly used in project management is a Gantt chart. (EMRs do not use Gantt charts for patients, but they are definitely built to support thinking that way, and I would like to illustrate a point.) If you are unfamiliar, a Gantt displays an engineered solution for navigating from the start of a project, at the upper left, to the end of the project, at the lower right. Tasks are listed down the side of the chart in the order they need to be done (i.e., according to their dependencies), dates are arrayed across the top, and bars within the grid cascade neatly along the path from inception to solution.

Now imagine a patient with heart disease and new onset diabetes. Our tasks would be, say, to control her lipids, sugars, and the ever-present obesity, and we woul like to get it done in the next 6 months. We are at Point A, we would like to get to Point B, and the Gantt maps the road ahead. Trivial.

Unfortunately, our road quickly gets bumpy. The vascular disease has reduced her kidney function and her ejection fraction, and so restricts our use of metformin or pioglitazone. Meanwhile, the patient feels "low" with her sulfonylurea, so she only takes it when she thinks she needs it. The resultant hyperglycemia gives us uncontrolled triglycerides, so our lipids are knocked off course. And by the way, the patient read something about the statin is killing her liver, so she stopped that one altogether. Her obesity is exacerbated because no calories are being delivered to her musculature, and it is further worsened by the growth hormone-like effects from her hyperinsulinemia. By week 4 she complains of hot flashes and remembers the chronic arthritis in her knee, and shortly she develops a MRSA-infected foot ulcer.

Our carefully engineered project is so far off course that, by midway, our Gantt chart has become pointless. It is more than just a deviation from our plotted course; we are getting saddled with new problems that may or may not be related to our original plan. Project management includes mishaps, of course, but we are experiencing a total meltdown, and this is routine in medicine.

With verbatim reasoning, our attempts to address each of our objectives have hit an insurmountable roadblock: "non-compliance." But with gist reasoning, new opportunities arise. Keeping the meaning of our work in mind, using intent alone to guide us, we abandon the sulfonylurea and the statin, and instead try celecoxib. On the surface, a COX-2 inhibitor has nothing to do with our project, and it might even introduce additional cardiac risk. (A verbatim no–no!) But when the patient's knee pain improves, she starts walking more, then her sugars stabilize, the triglycerides improve, the circulation to her foot helps heal it faster, her cardiac ejection fraction rises, and she feels more energetic and loses weight. Then, since I am just making this up, she abandons her sedentary lifestyle and achieves sustained health.

The reason we are treating this patient is to moderate her cardiovascular risk, among other things, and our use of celecoxib has helped achieve it. The reason does not provide a target per se, but rather a broad intention, which might find satisfactory expression as any of a number of targets. Elsewhere, such a cluster of possible targets has been called a "decision cloud," to distinguish it from the point-like destination implied by the lower right corner of the Gantt chart, and to hint that it requires a diffusion of the engineered path somewhere high in the chart, rather than a simple digression at the very end. A decision cloud is analogous to the quantum cloud of probabilities where an electron roams; when we finally look, our solution might have ultimately precipitated from anywhere within it.

EMRs as currently built cannot accommodate decision clouds, nor can practice guidelines. Yet we create those clouds every day by understanding and manipulating the meaning of our work. Any of a number of solutions might achieve our purpose, and maintaining our focus on intention, not just details, is how we dynamically navigate along many possible patient care trajectories.

An experienced clinician's decision-making is categorical and meaningful, often reflective of just those critical few determinants of divergence or convergence within a taxonomy of similar patients. It is not an assembly of isolated facts and a recitation of the entire possible decision tree (i.e., the differential diagnosis). This probably explains the frequently observed recession of progress note lengths in the written record: the verbatim-trained medical student writes two pages of disjointed facts, the resident, a page of more selective findings, the fellow, a paragraph of interpreted results, and the attending can capture the essence of the patient and the entire plan in just a couple of lines. That fact drives billing clerks and lawyers crazy, but as succinct as it is, the attending's note actually represents a completely reasoned medical decision. The completeness of that communication does, however, presume a reader with similar training and experience.

So, the fundamental reason that EMRs typically fail to *help* physicians stems from the disconnect between how we portray medical reasoning and how we actually perform it. EMRs are built for an idealized, deterministic, and literal vision of medical practice, which might be well-suited for the nascent clinician, but it is an impediment to the experienced professional.

I have spent a lot of time in this section sketching out the difference between what EMRs are designed to do and what we actually do. Understanding this is an essential first step for success. It is important to have a clear view of what EMRs can and cannot do, and the ways they can be expected to help and hinder our thinking, in order to best optimize our use of them.

I have provided some references at the end of this section to help you further understand your mindset, particularly for exploring Fuzzy Trace and sociotechnical systems. In the meantime, do not succumb to the EMR's native methods of patient management; it will frustrate you to no end. There are no paved roads yet, so try driving it off the beaten path. Reframe your frustrations. Rather than finding fault with the technology regard it as a problem of evolving and optimizing a complex sociotechnical system. Build hybrid solutions with paper and EMR processes working together. We have come full circle back to the laboratory: experiment, ruminate, and learn, then apply the feedback. And *be careful when deciding about spending excessive amounts of money* to try to solve a problem inherent to the system by seeking solutions from additional technical features.

Maintenance

This second section is where you work *for the EMR*. Sorry. But the best assistant you ever had was one you trained carefully and thoroughly. You are used to cultivating people, now you have to domesticate the EMR. It will eventually work for you. That, or you will pull its plug.

While the routine of maintenance is easily overlooked during your planning and implementation, it is important to realize that it takes real time and resources, and is critical to success. Surviving the initial asteroid blast does not automatically confer success during the winter that follows. In an institution, the roles and functions described below are doled out among multiple individuals, if not entire committees, but even in a solo practice each of them must be addressed.

Roles

Let us start with an overview of some of the key roles involved in EMR maintenance. These are the same roles utilized during concurrent optimization, but I will not repeat them in that section.

The Physician Champion/Super User/Problem Solver

In post-implementation surveys, the role most consistently cited as the reason for success is that of the physician champion or its variations. In an institution, this would map to the CMIO position. This person (or people) is the glue that holds the project together, and the role is probably summarized as performing physician liaison – between providers and technology, and also between providers and governance.

To be effective, the person must be part coach, part cheerleader, and part drill sergeant. He/she must be a respected clinician, must have sufficient resources available to be an effective trouble-shooter, must have a natural enthusiasm for not just the technology, but also for its success, and also must have adequate coping skills to avoid burn-out. It is a highly visible and hands-on role, not hidden in a cubicle – that is for the worker bee (below). He/she also needs sufficient authority to make decisions. While coordination through committees helps ensure vertical and horizontal integrity of the system and provides external validation for interim decisions, too many simple things get mired and lost in formal processes. The project will fail if it becomes too unresponsive to the ongoing needs of the users.

The physician champion performs many functions revolving around liaison: communicating process changes, managing expectations, relaying tips and discoveries among the various users, solving problems (both immediate and long-term), and directing service requests. One of the most successful ways to accomplish all those functions has been called the "Buddy-Blitz." This is when the super user/champion shadows a provider 1:1 for several days at a time, helping to tweak every aspect of the system as the provider is actually using it. A buddy-blitz might be routinely considered at go-live, but its best effect is when it is repeated episodically. It is very expensive (the super user is a clinician, remember) and time-intensive, but it can virtually guarantee buy-in to have users' settings personalized, favorites lists built, shortcuts demonstrated, and so on.

As the implementation stabilizes, the champion role evolves to assume many of the ongoing management functions delineated below, but there are three in particular which are paramount. First, this person has to develop an intense focus on clinical outcomes and objectives. He/she is a clinician to begin with, and EMRs expose patients to the possibility of unintended consequences and systematic harm (see Optimization below), and it is critical to have someone thinking about and monitoring the intersection of technology and patient care. Second, the champion has to advocate for providers. EMR implementations are done for myriad reasons, and they are not all convergent. Occasionally, what the providers need can directly compete with other project goals, such as operating cost savings. Implementations can fail for a million reasons, but one of the biggest is not supporting the providers. Third, the champion is the impetus for creatively adapting the EMR to the office ecosystem. This person straddles the technical and clinical worlds and is thereby best positioned to see the possibilities, tinker with alternatives, and re-structure some facet of the technology or culture. As I mentioned previously, this is an essential piece of the success puzzle and can well be the final determinant of success or failure.

I would like to make a final point. The champion role is either a physician or an extender. Your nurse or tech cannot perform it, not because they do not have the savvy or wherewithal, but because they have their own transformation going on, and their use of the EMR, even their particular screens, can be markedly different than those of the providers. Moreover, they should not be given access to your level of function within the system – beyond the medico-legal and audit trail issues that it would create, they may not be able to correctly address the ubiquitous alerts or messages. It is already a mine field; no need to make the EMR still more dangerous.

Thought Leaders/Early Adopters

During and after implementation, especially if there is a lot of push-back from users, it is helpful to identify providers who are already seen as thought leaders within the organization. They do not have to be super users or even particularly adept at the EMR; you just need their buy-in. They will form your critical mass during implementation and are well worth 1:1 engagement. Focus resources on them to encourage early adoption of whatever phase you are working on, and the rest often follow like dominoes. They also will ultimately take some of the burden off the champion role.

IT Worker Bees

These are the brave souls who actually make the project a success. They take their direction from governance and the champion and must have excellent working relationships with the providers (so they need both enthusiasm and thick skins). They work under the hood, building order sets and templates, and so on. This is such a pivotal role, staffing here often completely offsets any FTE gains the organization might have accumulated from reductions in paper filing or dictation. Even in small practices, this role needs to be filled.

Executive Governance

We can all intuit that competent governance makes or breaks a project, but somewhat surprisingly, this role is not often cited in the surveys of the most important features for success. But do not skimp on it, please. Governance during maintenance and optimization does evolve somewhat from the functions necessary during planning and implementation (see Chapter 4), and eventually supervises everything under "Functions" below.

Governance is usually driven by a committee. In a small practice it can be and probably should be everyone who touches the system. You will need every perspective to maintain the integrity of your entire sociotechnical system. The effectiveness of governance depends on balancing all the competing agendas. Every position takes a performance hit and gains some efficiencies, and it is among the duties of governance to distribute those costs and benefits. The committee also needs to have sufficient authority to enact changes without further confirmation, so decision-makers are an essential component.

A specific point about governance is that in larger organizations, it needs to be protected by peer review. That means it needs to have a permanent position within the organizational structure, and it means defining its charter in a way that avoids redundant authority. The need for peer review arises from the frank discussions that must occur when patient outcomes are concerned, and there must be a formal mechanism available to governance to intervene if necessary. This requirement also implies that non-clinical members of the committee might need to be dismissed during certain proceedings.

Functions

Now let us look at the work that needs to be done. A baker's dozen of items that require maintenance are reviewed here. They are not exhaustive but more illustrative of many facets that governance has to engage. While reviewing these functions, pay particular attention to how expensive they are, especially in terms of time and energy. Vendors never, and consultants only rarely, include these costs in their return on investment (ROI) analyses, and your HITECH stimulus will not even come close to covering them (see Optimization below).

Managing Cultural Changes

The implementation of an EMR represents a profound organizational transformation, and it is HARD to do. You are interfering with typically highly evolved work patterns. The cultural change for providers will be your biggest challenge, but staff will not be far behind.

With providers, start by aiming for just a critical mass of adoption – maybe 30–50% of your clinicians. Focus on the thought leaders, as stated above. Once the ball is rolling, momentum alone will pick up most others. Your ultimate target is probably only 85–90% adoption – there are some people that you will never capture, although it may surprise you who they turn out to be. They are the dinosaurs, though, and the rest of you are the furry little mammals on the ascendancy. On the other hand, do not be so dismissive that you cannot help an old dinosaurs who is considering a species change.

There are two specific types of provider worth mentioning. The first is the actively resisting "I'm not doing it" kind. Ignore them, it is just that simple. They may wave the banner of spokesman-for-the-common-man, but if my section above about mindset was at all helpful to you, you are already that spokesman, and the troops will rally to your frank assessments. Trying to work with actively resistant providers is like performing heroic measures in the ICU – very expensive, exhausting, and usually ultimately futile. Instead, just dole out your measured response, the disciplinary or financial penalties established in the P&Ps, and move on. They may come along eventually. If for some reason benign neglect is not an option here (e.g., the provider is your only partner or is an important thought leader in your organization), then approach that person as you would be the naysayer, described next.

The second provider type does deserve some consideration. This is the naysayer: "it's not working," or "why can't it do this?" A subtle difference from the active resister, but the difference is often sufficient to tip them to your favor, eventually. These providers often arise from a group who claim to have been excluded from the vendor and product selection process. It does no good to point out the 15 engraved invitations that were extended to them, but they had been "too busy." Instead, graciously accept that they were not part of the planning phase, put it behind you, and ask how you can help them move forward.

Inclusion is usually the answer here; now that you have got their full attention. Bring them into the fold and engage them in pilots or governance. These providers can make the EMR work a whole lot better for everyone; ask for their help. They will cost you a lot of personal collateral – including them can be bruising at first – but if you can score points with any of them, other naysayers will often come along too. Give them ample buddy-blitzing and learn from their requests.

With regard to all the other providers, they will have degrees of grumbling about various features or circumstances, but they do not usually revert to either of the two types described above. Keep them all engaged by working hard to personalize what you can. Creating personal order sets especially helps, but that is a double-edged sword. On the one hand, providers love tweaking them until they are just perfect for themselves, and any small achievements in efficiencies will help buy-in considerably. On the other hand, you have just frittered away your ability to standardize care and it may be harder than you think to get it back again.

When dealing with providers, present them with dispassionate data. Do not try to sugar coat or spin your way out of bad news, but rather describe your frank assessment and your plan to get through it. In particular, the providers are going to take a performance hit, and if they are paid on production, they are also going to take financial hit. Depending on the size of your initiative, you might need to have some form of compensatory payment during the implementation period. This is all the more important if the EMR is being driven by executive mandate. In addition, providers may also need to be paid for their time in assisting implementation or governance. It is also fair to demonstrate that improved efficiencies in one arena can offset the lost efficiencies that the providers are feeling most acutely.

The cultural changes for your staff are just as disruptive, although it just does not elicit nearly so much push back. I would maintain an evenhanded presentation to the staff, emphasizing inclusion and data in a similar way as with the providers. Their job descriptions will be subjected to a lot of refinement and redefinition, and their biggest concerns usually revolve around their employment status. If it is unlikely that the staff will be losing any jobs, I would present that first and repeat it often.

One final piece which becomes increasingly important over time is surviving staff turnover. As an EMR is implemented, a great deal of sociotechnical change occurs, and the particulars of how a position functions within the new context is usually not well known. That is, with so much job-specific learning going on, there is not much emphasis on cross-training. When a critical employee leaves, you risk losing a great deal of know-how that you paid for through both formal training and lost production. The best remedy to offset your risk is to secure that know-how shortly after the learning curve has flattened. Use that knowledge as training material for cross-over positions and archive it for ultimate knowledge recovery after staff turnover.

Managing Process Changes

If cultural change is the hardest thing you are going to do, process change is the most fundamental thing you have to do. There is very little intrinsic to an EMR which improves your efficiencies and outcomes. I will grant one concession here: the technology obviously allows for the patient chart to be in multiple places at once. Most of the gains in efficiency have nothing to do with the technology, but rather have to do with process reengineering.

The best way to approach process change is in the form of incremental experiments. Designed and redesigned processes are more likely to succeed when various incremental changes have been tested and proven reliable. In addition, incremental change helps considerably for staff buy-in, since they do not feel overwhelmed quite so easily.

Governance needs to manage and direct imperatives to change from multiple directions. You should be open to bottom-up recommendations from every position among your staff and providers. You will also need to respond to executive mandates for top-down changes. Additional imperatives come from certifying bodies, new research, changes in your business environment, and new opportunities.

Examples of process changes include the timing of bringing back a patient and how much is added to the chart prior to the provider seeing the patient. Additional workflows might change regarding how phone calls will be returned or how prescriptions will be refilled. One of the most obvious changes in process after EMR implementation is provider documentation.

One of the biggest selling points for patient safety is using computerized physician order entry (CPOE). Legibility is no longer an issue, and order sets help constrain orders to stay within specific parameters. Another advantage of computerized entry is that you can order from multiple venues including from home or while traveling. One large disadvantage is that much of the traditional workflow for executing an order is returned squarely to the provider's shoulders. Some measurements have shown a sevenfold increase in the amount of time it takes a provider to construct an order with an EMR. Take note of that number.

One other modified process with clear implications for the EMR is coding and billing. My advice in this arena is to proceed very cautiously. Medicare in particular is scrutinizing the EMR's ability to cut and paste documents together, and even when the EMR is being used according to its intent, you may be vulnerable to allegations of fraud.

Whatever changes in workflow are going to occur, one of the best techniques I have found for planning and educating is to use an organizing rubric called "start-stop-continue." The concept is simple: for every change, specify what new features are being started, which previous features are being stopped, and which features continue unchanged.

I have one last observation about process change during the transition to the EMR. Your priorities will be different depending on what your processes were prior to the EMR. If you are coming from all paper, the tendency is to emphasize the presence of workstations and printers, the physician champion, and the new workflows. On the other hand, if you are changing from a previous EMR, the tendencies are to emphasize technical training, technical support, and security and privacy issues, while not spending nearly so much time with workflow modification.

Managing the Vendor (Technical Support)

There is an old Taoist paradox that notes that the utility of a wheel comes from the emptiness in the middle, namely, where the axle is placed. I recognize that wheel. We beg for scraps and at the table, while a trillion dollar industry swirls around us. The imaging, the laboratories, the medical equipment, the pharmaceuticals, and yes, the software, all cannot exist without our orders and without our patients. There must be a tremendous centrifugal force that sends the money flying out to the perimeter – the profit margins are huge among the healthcare support industries when compared to the healthcare provision industry. No doubt primary care, if not the whole of medical practice, is the utility in the middle of the healthcare wheel.

EMR vendors profit considerably from their work. Most vendor markups are on the order of a 100% profit. The methods by which vendors make their money usually fall into two camps, and neither is especially good for us. In the first camp, they make their money predominantly by selling installations; these vendors often do not cultivate a strong support service, especially for older EMR versions, and that will eventually leave you up the proverbial creek. In the second camp, they make their money mostly by providing support; they charge an arm and a leg for it up front, then they charge additional appendages for the piece work that comes later. While I am capitalist enough to believe that profit is not wholly immoral, profiteering surely is. Non-clinical costs are the fastest rising segment of our national healthcare expenditures.

The costs for EMR technical support typically range from $1000 to $20,000 per physician per year, depending on what you buy. Training and technical support are usually provided during the implementation phase by the original contract. Meanwhile, you will need it in an ongoing fashion, and that is negotiated separately. My only specific recommendation is to read your contracts carefully and ask a lot of questions. Help may also be available online, and some may be very specific to your EMR, in the form of online forum communities. Other tips might come from a nearby practice where the same EMR has also been implemented. Be on the lookout for freebies among those venues.

The primary aim in contracting for technical support is to create a partnership. Your relationship to the vendor should be similar to that of a marriage. Too often support issues degenerate into a shouting match regarding who owns the problem; get away from "my problem versus their problem," instead it is always "our problem." In assembling your specific contract, link your successes together. Note that vendors are going to start with a shelf contract, but it is all negotiable, especially given that they are making a considerable amount of money on you. One strategy is to pay the first installment of their annual support fee only after the users cross a certain threshold for, say, order entry or online documentation. Even better, pay their money after you see a return on yours, especially if that was one of their selling points (see the Optimization section below).

You have more leverage than you think when negotiating contracts. The market for ambulatory EMRs is completely under-penetrated, as mentioned in the Chapter introduction above. Use the DesRoches data to do some calculations: there are between 500,000 and 750,000 physicians engaged in active patient care in the US. Four percent of that means there are 20,000–30,000 physicians using a full EMR and 13% means there are 65,000–95,000 using a partial EMR. And that is the *entire* installed base so far. When your vendor says they are servicing so many gazillion doctors, call them out on it. If the sales representative who is working with you on your contract does not seem to understand, move up the line. Seek management level intervention and point out that success with you may cascade into successes with other ambulatory practices in your community or even elsewhere. If by the time you are reading this you have already signed your contract, try to renegotiate it – any vendor who wants a piece of that huge open market wants your business, and by the way, other vendors would love to steal your business away from their competitor.

A final point about managing your vendor arises from the potential for disagreement over who owns what within the EMR. The end-user license agreement (EULA) is a nonnegotiable contract: you must consent to it before you can actually use any software. This puts you on unequal footing with the vendor, and you may have no recourse. When you think you have created the world's perfect order set or template for patient care, most EULAs hold that the work belongs to the vendor, since you used the vendor's software to build them. You agreed to the EULA and have little recourse.

Your best strategy is to document everything you have done yourself, so that at least the knowledge will transfer if you need to abandon your vendor and the EMR. That documentation can also save you if the vendor is bought out or goes under, both of which are still happening with considerable frequency in the industry. For example, McKesson's entire EMR product line is assembled out of acquisitions of smaller vendors. The problem with this process is that your EMR's new management may have different priorities regarding your particular product; you may be left high and dry with an unsupported or archaic EMR. Documentation of processes, policies, order sets, etc. will form your safety net.

Managing Service Requests

Service requests (SRs) formalize the many calls for changes or repairs to the system that arise from the end users, and they represent the form that exchanges take under your technical support contract. Some requests fall within your own control, but many fall to the vendor. It is the task of governance to prioritize and route these requests, and occasionally generate strategic requests of its own, usually to steer the overarching objectives for the system.

A particular set of services that governance often generates is the request for interfaces with or uploads from other systems, needed to realize optimal EMR effectiveness. These services are usually negotiated as line items on your support contract, and they can be very expensive, since they often need to be custom built (due to the absence of national standards). For example, you may be interested in connecting with specific hospitals, other practices, or local pharmacies; you may also be very interested in uploading data from old practice management software or legacy systems. These services may be particularly important at the institutional level, where you likely have a considerable investment in the old data.

Despite the expense, merging old data into your new system has the potential to pay for itself, by reducing re-work and by fleshing out patient data. At our hospital we noticed a precipitous drop in our patient case mix after implementing our new EMR. We had inadvertently dropped many of the diagnoses that patients had carried from encounter to encounter in the old system. Once these older diagnoses were ported into the new patient charts, our case mix returned to its previous levels.

Managing service requests usually starts with collecting problems during particular scenarios. When a problem arises, you need to capture as much of the surrounding circumstance as possible, including which user was involved, what was being attempted, what screen was being viewed, and even which specific patient chart was active at the time. Accumulate the scenarios, and patterns will emerge, and those patterns will focus your resulting service requests.

The SRs themselves need to be tracked very carefully. Spreadsheets or mini databases can help considerably. First, keep the original scenarios attached to their associated SR, so they can later become the basis for your test scripts after the SR has been completed. That is, you recreate the original scenario and make sure that the SR has adequately addressed the problem.

Second, since there is neither money nor time to fix everything, use the SR database to set priorities, and schedule the work to be done. In general, push complaints and suggestions from your providers to the top, since the new workflows fall heavily to them, and if they fail, so does the EMR.

Third, track the progress of each SR, including who owns the problem, since not all of them need to be routed through the vendor. If the SR does belong to the vendor, assign a member of your own team to push it through. It is more than just becoming a squeaky wheel, although that definitely helps. You can actually negotiate the timeline of high priority SRs with the vendor, and it may not even cost you extra if you can find in your support contract any language that implies that the responsibility was the vendor's to begin with.

Lastly, create a flagging system within your SR database for problems that present risks to patient care. These SRs require special attention; you need a rapid response to them. That must include immediate intervention so the problem cannot be replicated while the fix is in process. One of the implications here is that the champion and IT worker bees need sufficient authority to intercede without waiting for the formality of a governance committee meeting.

In summary, your objective is to create a tight process for continually improving and tweaking your EMR, and carry that process forward with you. Part of it should include a closed feedback loop to the end users who noticed a problem in the first place – it creates a great image of responsiveness and effectiveness and conveys the fact that we are all working to the same end. After an SR has been completed and the correction is deployed, a new education and training cycle ensues (see below). Finally, monitor the results; if the correction has unintended consequences, your process should include retrieving and implementing a roll-back position.

Managing Incremental Roll-Outs

There are many ways to roll out an EMR. The Big Bang approach generates the most resistance but guarantees all the parts of the system come up together and interrelate their data correctly. The approach that is relevant for maintenance and optimization is the incremental roll-out. This style generates the heaviest load on project administration, but it allows roll-back of failed segments, it smoothes cultural transitions, and can allow some incremental recovery of investment before proceeding to new phases. Its downsides include the possibility that it perpetually delays completion of the project, and it shifts issues of global security, reliability, and interoperability onto the owner and away from the vendor.

During incremental roll-out, governance has a number of options available to phase in features. One is to create formal phases – I, II, III, etc. – which amount to Mini Bangs. What helps most here is to disconnect the twin timelines of development and deployment; that is, build your new features completely offline, then simply choose when to activate them. A less formal technique than phasing is to make processes only partially mandatory. For example, all H&Ps and Discharge Summaries have to be done in the system, but progress notes can be straight dictated. Note, however, that leaving an "out" to your providers may undermine their motivation to master the learning curve.

A favorite alternative to either phases or partial mandates is to implement a feature with a pilot group first. You gain the advantage of working out some kinks before widespread dissemination, but your enthusiastic pilot group might not be critical enough to truly assess the weak spots, and double deployment means virtually double the work. A variation, really a hybrid with partial mandates, is to turn a feature on for everyone, designate a pilot group to focus on testing it, but allow anyone else to join in as soon as their interest stirs. You will attract tinkerers and toe-dippers, but will avoid the more confrontational style of mandates, and with luck, you might even accumulate a critical mass of adoption with minimal effort.

Managing Forms, Templates, and Order Sets

These parts of the EMR usually represent the customizable features that are completely under your control. This is where any of the benefits to patients would occur, that is, if clinical outcomes turn out to be amenable to management by controlling variation in practice (so far, the research literature suggests otherwise). This is also where process efficiencies can be gained with semi-automation of the rote portions of our work.

Forms, templates, and order sets all need to blend clinical objectives and operational efficiencies with understandable presentations and are often best designed by an interested multidisciplinary team. The force that competes with this recommendation is that of encouraging EMR adoption through personalized provider preferences. It is up to governance to find the balance; it will no doubt lean toward the individual preferences, for its incentive effect, early during implementation, then migrate toward more organization-wide uniformity later. Governance will have to shepherd that migration and track and fuse proliferating versions. As with SRs, a mini database can be helpful here, for tracking versions and the cascades of document dependencies (e.g., which forms will need rebuilding after a particular change in the formulary).

When engaging your multidisciplinary team, recognize that it is expensive time. Stay focused on chronic conditions with high occurrence rates in your practice, especially if there are disease guidelines readily available (do not re-invent the wheel) and if performance measures are established or likely in the near future. Within the team, it usually works best if there is a point person or sponsor of a particular form or template. This person collates ideas, advocates for changes, and manages progress. They also chair the ad hoc committees used to create specific content for their charges.

Many EMRs allow for collapsible/explodable forms. This feature is usually applied to the hierarchical nature of physical exam findings, and collapsing a form can help keep the final document reasonably readable and relevant. The down side is that many clicks are necessary to explode a hierarchy so you can find what you are looking for, and a fully expanded form can be many pages long. Eventually, users remember where in the hierarchy various things are, but until then, minimize the depth of the collapsing features.

A variation of the collapsing form concept is the branching of order sets and protocols. This kind of feature needs to be designed and experimented with carefully. There are several things to balance. The more an order set branches, the more flexible it becomes, the broader its scope, and the less likely something is overlooked. They can do quite a bit of work for your providers. On the other hand, branching orders imply an attempt to manage patients with multiple conditions, patients in this population tend to be very complicated, and their care is often intrinsically resistant to protocols. Like collapsing forms, branching sets also take many more clicks to navigate, and they require intensive attention to maintain them.

Even simple order sets have their balance points. To be helpful, most individual orders need to be as nearly complete as possible, but the more complete an order is, the less widely applicable it becomes. Also, pre-selected items within option lists can achieve slam dunk status for performance indicators, but can unintentionally create inappropriate orders for patients too. It is again up to governance to find the balance. Governance also needs to supply the necessary policies to support automatic orders, such as having nurses dispense vaccinations to patients meeting certain criteria.

Very little consideration appears to ever be given to the arrangement and display of information in documents and reports. We are a document-centric culture – that is, the artifacts of our patient encounters are the documents we create. We specifically sign them to signify that a given document represents an integrated unit of observations, interpretations, and decisions. EMR developers may have missed some of the nuance of our documents. They spend enormous energy finding ways to capture data, but rarely create good tools for designing its retrieval and presentation – the black hole model I mentioned earlier. All the data is there, but the reports generated by EMRs have all the elegance of a data dump. Moreover, since developers do not often know what kind of questions we will ask of our data or which performance metrics we will want to track, they do not create any sophisticated tools for data mining or analysis. The effort it used to take to calculate your dashboard indicators by hand is nearly matched by the effort it will take to retrieve their electronic cousins. It takes digging, refining, re-formatting, and cross-checking before output data is useful.

So governance also has to spend time and energy designing the forms and templates and data sources for reports. And like so much else with your EMR, it is hard work and is definitely not a simple byproduct of using the system. But if insufficient care is taken here, your providers will revert to paper notes and marginalia so they can actually think about their patients, and management will be grasping for understandable trends, or worse, making decisions based on incomplete or erroneous data.

A final function of governance regarding forms, templates, and order sets is their ultimate retirement. When forms are updated, flawed, not being used correctly, or not being used at all, it is time to archive them and delete them from the system. At best they create unnecessary clutter; at worse they dangerously redirect the flow of patient care.

Managing Policies and Procedures

P&Ps are probably familiar territory if you have participated in governance of any kind. The introduction of an EMR into your organization presents opportunities to review and revise P&Ps to reflect the new technology and processes. Important changes to existing policies need to be taught right alongside the new features of the EMR.

An EMR brings the requirement for entirely new policies too. One requirement is to specify what goes into a provider's inbox, and who can gain access to it. You might direct timing-sensitive messages to a "all-comers" type inbox or copy those messages to every capable provider, so that if the provider who was the original destination for the message is unavailable, someone else can provide backup.

Alternatively, you could restrict any timing-sensitive material from entering the message queue at all, and instead direct it to a tracking board type function. Even when a message is not particularly timing-sensitive, it still might become critical if it sits in an inbox for a week while a provider is away. The away provider can grant a proxy for another person to access his/her inbox while away, but the policy covering that method has to emphasize that the designee then has the responsibility to act on the messages, not just read them.

Since communication breakdown is one of the critical dangers during and after EMR implementation, you might choose none of the above options, and instead continue your previous process of verbally transmitting important messages. It is one of the more bizarre scenes among all of the EMR transformations, watching people who previously bantered casually and exchanged information freely, now all intensely glued to their monitors and quietly tapping on keyboards. A little bit of retro policy here can dislodge them and recreate the esprit de corps that we know engenders excellence, no matter what the venue.

Another specific area to create new policies is regarding the redistribution of the workload. EMRs place enormous loads on the providers to chart, to order, to bill, to reconcile, and to continue to care for patients – functions which had previously been arrayed across a whole office full of staff. Providers can delegate some responsibilities to a less expensive and less overwhelmed person who is still competent to perform the function, especially when guided by a clear policy.

Yet another new area for policy is that of specifying naming conventions. It might seem too trivial to formally address, but as patient documents, templates, forms, reports, order sets, and so on, proliferate over the years, it will become nearly impossible to find what you are looking for without some rules. Within a year of go-live at my hospital, we had an even dozen stroke protocols – for the ED, for the rapid response team, for the ICU, and so on. It is not so important what form the final rules take, just that they are simple enough to remember, both for saving and for retrieving documents. Since most EMR lists are alphabetical by default, make sure that documents you would like to cluster together all start with the same words.

For example, everything to do with a particular patient can be named [last name]_[first name]_[MI]_[date of birth]_[date of service]_[document type]_[provider name, if available], and so on. If a large collection of documents from many patients were in a directory, alphabetical sorting would readily cluster all of a single patient's documents together with a sub-clustering by date of service. Which patient you need and the approximate date of service are among the most common items you know when you are looking for something. In larger institutions, you might need to include service unit names, or create a specialty cluster before the document type. You could start every template's name with the body system it applies to such as cardiac or pulmonary, which disease such as diabetes, or which venue in an institution such as telemetry.

In addition to naming the documents, policies need to specify what types of document belong where within the system. Are cath reports from an outside institution placed in an "Outside Documents" folder or a "Cardiac" folder? Are telephone calls saved under "Telephone Calls" or under "Progress Notes," since events during the phone call can shape the next office visit? In the paper chart, such distinctions are not always drawn, and notes of all kinds often flow continuously through the record. But the EMR is more rigidly structured, and governance needs to set out how to impose that structure.

Other policies might be needed to address who owns the medication reconciliation process in any given setting or when a correction is allowed to document and when an addendum is required instead. Many of the other functions of governance itemized above and below will also need policies to support them. More work, more expense, very little support by your vendor, and none of these costs are recognized by our legislators.

Managing Education, Training, and Support

Whenever and wherever change arises, it requires new education to implement it. If done well, education materials can be a form of captured organizational knowledge, but they need to be constantly synchronized with process and policy changes. Maintaining these materials requires a focused and enduring effort. There is a balance: a comprehensive indexed reference is invaluable, but heavily documented (read: cumbersome) training manuals will not be read.

Teaching for providers is generally most effective when the teaching is scenario based. The best method is to balance a scripted clinical scenario with free exploration within the EMR. Combining real patients' redacted charts is the best source material, since real records guarantee at least some internal consistency among the labs, the orders and so on. Generally, teach one best way to perform a function in the EMR, even if there are many ways or shortcuts. Those will come with time to those who are interested. Also, as mentioned above, teach the new policies and procedures alongside the new technology.

Providers do best with one-on-one teaching. I suppose it can be embarrassing (even crippling) for a doctor to be a respected authority in professional life but struggling to use the computer during training. If your format starts with one-on-one, rather than defaults to it for someone who is struggling, you will deftly sidestep this problem and encourage buy-in, especially among your senior physicians. Since providers ultimately only learn the system when they actively use it, the buddy-blitz often turns out to be the best implementation of this strategy, even though it is expensive.

Managing Security and Compliance

Many of the governance functions listed thus far cost a lot, but much of that money is being spent on yourself and your staff, so you could conceivably count it as an investment, although it will not bring much of a financial return. With regard to compliance, however, entire outside industries have been spawned to help us conform to HIPAA, Joint Commission, Medicare, Leap Frog, and so many other rules and recommendations. Incidentally, the new HITECH Act, described in more detail in the next section, adds considerably more teeth to issues of security and privacy than HIPAA had.

So much advice about security and compliance has been bought, that we have returned again to the Taoist wheel – our own healthcare dollars spiraling away from us empty folks in the center. Why do Eastern philosophies prize emptiness so much? While you ponder that one, I will keep my remarks here focused on just three issues, since so much expensive opinion on compliance has already come before me.

The first issue regards the security and privacy problems surrounding electronic health data. You would think that security would be a relatively easy feature for the vendor to produce, as compared to the intellectual gymnastics necessary to care for a patient, for example. But too many vendors only think of security after they have built their EMRs, and bolt-on versions are sieves compared to security built into the software from the ground up. Since we are the professionals who actually use these systems, we bear the brunt of responsibility for privacy and security, not our vendors. This responsibility is amplified if you have assembled your EMR out of components.

Study how to use audit trails and use them regularly. While it is true that audit trails are reactive, spot checking them is a little like a beat cop walking around his neighborhood. You have to assume that your security plan is not perfect and spend time detecting aberrations. Additionally, while it is a big provider selling point to do some charting or ordering from home, remote access introduces a number of risks, so take your time in designating what kind of access is available to your EMR. Finally, many security threats and privacy violations unfortunately come from within your own organization, so look for the ability to create tiered levels of security, design them carefully, and apply them to your users thoroughly. The short of it is to find the security features of your EMR and use them, even if you know they are imperfect. Most intrusions are opportunistic.

The second issue is one of compliance with performance metrics. There may be literally 500 indicators that you will ultimately be asked to track and report, and your EMR has at best just generic reporting abilities. You will have to dig for that data and test it, making sure you did no't miss some contributing sources or include some erroneous sources and making sure that the data ultimately makes sense. Incentives will be tied to reporting (see the comments on the HITECH Act next section), and unfortunately, even with an EMR, it will take considerable effort to do so accurately.

The final issue is another compliance note, one that returns to our infamous EULA. These unnegotiated contracts force you to deviate from Joint Commission requirements to protect patients from undue harm or to inform them if they face risk. Most EULAs require that you *not* disclose any known defects of the software, and they also have "hold harmless" clauses that protect the vendor from responsibility for bad outcomes, even if you were using the product exactly as designed. While private practice may not be held to JC requirements, think hard about the implications for our legal and ethical obligations to our patients. We took an oath; our vendors did not.

Managing Down-Time

OK, so there are not any sophisticated bumper stickers that say "Down-time happens." But it sure does happen, and when it does, it feels a lot like what the other, related, bumper sticker. And worst of all, we still have to see the patients, no matter what is "happening."

There are three kinds of down-time that governance must manage: scheduled, unscheduled, and catastrophic. I do not usually consider sluggish performance to be a form of down-time, but if it were truly impeding patient care, then it would probably map to unscheduled down-time.

What happens during down-time is driven by P&Ps. The first step is to set thresholds, perhaps different for each of the three types, for what to do with data while the system is unavailable. For example, if it's down for 2 hours or less, re-enter the data when it comes back up; if it is down for more than that, handle down-time work like you would papers from outside the organization (e.g., scan them in, or maintain a paper record for them and place a reference in the electronic chart).

The processes while the system is unavailable might revert to those from before the EMR, or they might mirror the EMR processes entirely, just using paper versions of the screens to record patient data. As with most problems facing governance, the best solution is usually a balance of features from both approaches. Since down-time is P&P driven, each staff member should know what they are expected to do, and there should be no need for panicked calls to support about what to do, unless it is just to notify them of the problem.

Disaster recovery, from an event such as Katrina, is planned separately, but it usually takes the form of an extended version of unscheduled down-time. Regularly scheduled full backups and intermittent partial backups, somewhere off site, are necessary, but if the disaster hits your vendor, your safety net is yet again your paper trail. Keep a clear and complete archive of all your forms, processes, training materials, etc., and keep them safe. I might have mentioned you are not going to abandon paper, and that is the perfect segue to the next function of governance.

Managing Paper Parts of the Record

I do not think going paperless should be a target of EMR implementations. It is just too inefficient.

I have been trying to emphasize that EMRs are closer to snake oil than a cure for all of healthcare's ills, despite what Congress has been led to believe. What we are really trying to do, for the sake of patient care and fiscal responsibility, is to improve our processes and, perhaps, evolve a bit of symbiosis with information technology. A whole lot of things need to evolve before EMRs can become truly helpful, and until then, I say try to use the EMR for maybe 85% of your patient care functions, and leave that last 15% for better days ahead. Paper continues to work just fine for those knotted, irregular cases that just will not succumb to electronic straight-jackets.

Governance needs to manage paper parts of the record, from storing old practice records to receiving outside reports to generating pre-op H&Ps for outside specialists to filling in disability papers. Policies must be created for managing those artifacts, so it will not be much more complicated to include a few other processes chosen to remain paper-based, and the result can be liberating. For example, medication reconciliation at our hospital is disastrous when done with the EMR, so we bypass that functionality and use paper instead. By divorcing ourselves from one particularly inefficient part of the EMR, we not only regained our efficiencies, but we also staved off an open revolt from the internists. The policy might only be to scan all papers and shred them, but just thinking about a paper process will free you from rigidly applying the EMR to everything you have to get done, even if it performs very poorly at some of those functions.

The one set of papers that I would not shred, or at least would keep their scans completely separate from your EMR at all times, is your system and process documentation. This work has been bought and paid for by your own blood, sweat, and tears, and it is how you recover your old system or rebuild a new one when everything has gone horribly wrong.

Managing Upgrades

In the information technology industry, there is a classic conflict between working hard to maintain and support your existing products, or being responsive to changing requirements and possibilities and working hard to remake your products. Most software developers lean toward the latter and prefer to issue upgrades. There are different types of upgrades: some are periodic full version upgrades, some are interim patches to minor problems, and some are shameless extortion. Microsoft Word from 10 years ago works almost exactly the same as Microsoft Word from more recent years, yet people keep upgrading to the newer versions.

There are a few risks to ignoring upgrades. Specifically, your version may contain a dangerous flaw or vulnerability, or your version may no longer be supported. Likewise, there are risks (besides extortion) of implementing an upgrade, especially a major one for your EMR. These might include shutting the system down for some time to install the upgrade, disrupting yet again your well-honed processes, or finding that old data is now unreadable. It is very discouraging to perform an upgrade at the recommendation of your vendor, and only later find that something which worked well before now works horribly, or does not work at all.

There is a more insidious problem with upgrades to your EMR. All of the custom work that you did, creating templates and the like, have to be remade in the new system. Many times this is as simple as a cut and paste operation, but sometimes entire entities need to be rebuilt from scratch. Unfortunately, it is usually the most complicated branching order sets or nested templates that need rebuilding. Governance needs to choose which upgrades should be adopted, and how often, and balance having a better product against all that work to rebuild your customizations.

Testing and retesting are paramount while managing upgrades to your EMR. Any significant change to your system requires a 10-step cycle: (1) Develop a test plan. Stick to realistic patient scenarios as best you can. (2) Install the upgrade in your test environment. (3) Perform testing within the module of the EMR that was affected. (4) Perform integration testing between modules. Use your staff and have them represent their usual roles while playing out the patient scenarios. Have them test old problems to see if they have been fixed, have them check frequently used functions to see if they have been disrupted, have them look for weaknesses in the new version, and so on. (5) Design and document the affiliated process change. (6) Perform a system walk-through. Use your providers walk through entire processes. Do not evaluate your *designs* for features; rather, evaluate their actual implementation on the screen. (7) Educate and train users. (8) Backup your production system and create a restore point. (9) Install the upgrade in your production environment. (10) Conclude with documentation regarding things like why the change was necessary, what specifically did change, what forms or templates were affected and updated, which are now archived and obsolete, and any significant observations that arose out of the testing cycle.

One final point is to make sure that your testing and production environments stay synchronized. This is especially important if you accumulate many changes over time. If you installed a minor upgrade to your testing environment but never implemented it in production, the next major upgrade may perform completely differently during the testing cycle than when it is finally deployed. The point of testing is to mimic reality in every possible way, just short of actual patient care.

Managing Your Documentation

I have been emphasizing the paper trail created by all the functions of governance, over and above papers that belong to patient charts. I will try not to belabor the point, but these documents capture your organizational knowledge – clinical styles and business objectives and hard-won process efficiencies. Archive them carefully, be clear about which versions are current, and note where one document depends on another. The collection needs to have central management but also peripheral distribution for ready access during down-time. As mentioned elsewhere, a mini database can help keep track and the documents themselves can be deployed on an intranet, although be sure that they will not go down too when the system itself does.

Optimization

Optimization and improvement are done iteratively, meaning they are accomplished using repeated cycles. They are performed concurrently with maintenance functions, using the same roles. I think I might have mentioned that once you are using the EMR, the real work begins. Do not despair, we will get you there.

Optimization determines which side of the razor's edge of success you will fall onto. It is also where the most common reasons for buying an EMR are played out. (I will flag the top five as we come to each of them.) Recall the high EMR failure rates and realize that if left alone, the EMR will accomplish none of what you want from it. Like everything else I have discussed, optimization requires active management. It is, then, the final item in that long list of governance functions from the Maintenance section above. It is just so important that it gets a separate chapter.

Optimizations are similar to upgrades – both are meant to improve your system. The difference is that upgrades are driven by your vendor's agenda and optimization is driven by your own. This is the phase where you take control of this tool that has been little more than a task master since you acquired it. There are not any paved roads yet, so you can take it where you would like.

Optimization has its own 10-step cycle, somewhat different than the test cycle of upgrades, and more derivative of performance improvement methodologies. (1) Identify opportunities for enhancement, such as new functionality, functionality being underutilized, inefficient functions that need to be done in a different way, or just good old fashioned patient care initiatives. (2) Establish benchmarks by determining what data is going to be useful and how it should be presented. (3) Measure your current performance. (4) Establish goals and analyze the gaps. (5) Redesign the customizable parts of the EMR to fit your goals. (6) Redesign the surrounding workflow. (7) Design your change management strategy and educate affected staff. (8) Implement the change. (9) Measure your new performance, compare targets and outcomes, solicit feedback, and re-evaluate periodically for ongoing validity and relevance. (10) Document and archive this cycle.

You can contract for consultants to help you optimize your system. Sometimes you really just need outside help, for example, to nudge a cultural resistance problem along. But in many ways, this is more likely to be a waste of money. I have seen a well-known IT company advertising that its optimization services average a 30% increase in "beneficial system functionality." What is *that*? That they got you to turn on some meaningless bell or whistle? It is definitely *not* an ROI measure. Most of the things that consultants come up with, your champion could have told you, or would have figured out if he/she were not so harried all the time.

There are three basic components to optimization: technical, clinical, and financial.

Technical Optimization

There are about a thousand parameters that need to be tweaked in order to prevent your system's performance from becoming an issue. Their settings usually fall to the computer geeks. Initially, you will rely more on those settings directly associated with your vendor, but eventually you will rely mostly on your own local network technician. For example, your vendor will help set up the system so partial backups occur frequently enough that the most data you would ever lose from a power glitch might be limited to the last 15 minutes. Meanwhile your network technician will help keep the system fast enough that it always takes less than a second to respond to each mouse click. Technical optimization is an ongoing process, but most aspects should require your time only in the form of overarching governance.

One technical feature that needs specific direction from governance is device planning. This is more than just the number and placement of computer workstations; it also includes what kind of devices your system will support. While the vendor's product might have some limitations itself, more commonly you are deciding among the trade-offs involved for using wireless BlackBerries, hand-held tablet PCs, or sound cards and microphones to permit voice recognition. My recommendation is to accommodate your providers' preferences as much as your budget and available expertise will allow.

One other optimization that needs your attention is managing click-throughs. Let me explain. If your providers are using a feature for almost every encounter, you need to make sure that it takes a minimum number of clicks to get to that feature and get it done. This is obviously limited by what changes the software will allow, but working with your vendor (using service requests), you might be surprised at what you can streamline or provide shortcuts for. Focus especially on optimizing things you use 80% of the time; the remaining 20% are just going to take a few more clicks to complete.

Optimizing Clinical Outcomes

Improved patient safety and clinical outcomes represent the number one reason that EMRs are purchased, and should always be at the forefront of your mind as you use your EMR. Back to that oath we took. Before we look at optimization for patient care, I want to draw a distinction. I would say that a mistake is abnormal behavior, while an error is an abnormal result of normal behavior. The first comes from people or things doing something wrong; the latter is inherent to methods or systems. Both arise in patient care, but new ones arise from EMR use. There are arguments that patient harm from an EMR has more to do with suboptimal implementations than from use of the EMR per se. That argument is one of semantics only, as implementation problems are part and parcel of EMR problems.

EMRs start by obscuring where mistakes can arise. Before your EMR, if a patient care mistake occurred, it was usually either a misinterpretation or a frank mistake in judgment. With the EMR, those two problems can still occur, but now other mistakes can as well. It could be that you were not using the software correctly (this is the default position of your technical support). Or it could be that you were using it correctly, and it was functioning as intended, but the poor design has mismatched your expectations (i.e., the EMR is not doing what you think it should: this is often the real problem). Or it could be that you were using it correctly, and design was not the issue, but the system was not operating correctly. And the real problem with all of these is that you will be utterly lost trying to discern which mistake is actually creating the detected problem.

That more than doubles the number of ways a mistake can occur, but that is only the beginning. There are now a whole multitude of ways available to jeopardize patients, arising from new errors lurking within the immature sociotechnical system that we have tossed you and your staff into. If patient care was one of your top reasons to acquire an EMR, you need to actively manage these new risks.

One systematic error that can arise is the faltering of communication among team members. Recall the image of everyone quietly tapping on keyboards. Even without the banter, we often used to communicate with sticky notes, but now there is no place to put them. It takes a long time for everyone to get used to communicating via the EMR message center functions, and even then it seems a poor replacement for the immediacy and clarity of talking to someone, even if informally. This was one of the root causes of the increased ICU mortality that followed a CPOE implementation at Children's Hospital of Pittsburg [1].

Another error, one that also turned up at Pittsburg, is that EMRs can erect a cumbersome barrier to urgent and emergent care. They tend to distract providers' attention away from patients and more toward the workstations. Distraction can also occur in non-emergent office settings. For example, use caution when pressing providers to increase their encounter billing using the EMR features, because while the provider is trying to check everything off, he/she might totally miss the gist of the patient presentation.

Surprisingly, there are published reports of computerized order entry actually facilitating and perpetuating medication errors, which is the exact opposite of what it is supposed to do. For example, it can happen when the EMR carries forward an old amoxicillin prescription from last year. Because the patient never came back to have it "reconciled" off the record, a provider might opt not to treat a new tooth abscess, wanting instead to see how well the now long-expired antibiotic will work.

The EMR can hide information in plain sight, lost among copious irrelevant data. It also will not tell you if specific information is missing when there is so much other data to look at, and it can perpetuate erroneous information because it looks so convincing whenever a computer displays data.

Your overall approach to systematic error has got to be a systematic search for and flushing out of unintended consequences. Notice in particular that if you simply automate processes that had been poorly performed before the EMR, now you will automatically get that same poor performance every single time. And like politics, all quality is local – that is, quality improvement is a specialized reaction to the local intersection of issues that affect healthcare.

There are two methods for clinical optimization directly available to most EMRs. The rest of patient care improvement has to come from your mindset.

Decision Support

For most EMRs, decision support comes in the form of alerts, reminders, and guidelines. Be gentle here. The now famous revolt at Cedars-Sinai in Los Angeles was over too many "Are you sure?" interruptions while trying to order medications [2]. Notice that just having more information available, especially if its presentation is well-considered, can improve decisions right off the bat. So do not force too many decision support features; instead, accept a slow convergence onto best practices. Feedback, rather than directives, usually work best for guiding providers.

Alerts can flag interactions or contraindications. They are often limited to medications and allergies, and not disease processes. Their downside is that they lead to alert fatigue, which is when they pop up so frequently that they are dismissed reflexively, before they are even read. Acceptance of the information from an alert has been shown to be dependent on its clinical relevance; however, it is hard to find the right level of alert so that they are all relevant. To find out what level of alert works best for your providers, use the EMR itself to track how fast an alert is dismissed. If the average time is shorter than the time it takes to read one, you have got too many alerts. Many people eventually turn alerts off altogether, except maybe for the major interactions of medications. At our hospital, we route a lot of the alerts to the pharmacist instead of the physician.

Reminders help the most when you are trying to achieve benchmarks in performance or accreditation metrics. They are especially effective when coupled with policies and pre-selected orders within the EMR. They also help with health maintenance and preventive medicine tasks and can trigger follow ups for reviewing results or asking patients to come in.

Guidelines and clinical pathways can be customized and built for specific providers or specific patient populations (either diseases or demographics). There is a perennial and growing literature about their limitations, but they represent our best opportunity to standardize care on best practices. Within an EMR, they are assemblies of templates and/or order sets. I would recommend annotating them fully, because if a provider is looking at a guideline, there is a hint here that he/she might be searching for help, so use the moment to educate. In the end, the most refined guidelines in the world still require the clinician to determine its applicability. The only data we have to inform us about guideline design are studies that show suggestions or interventions for clinical decisions are rarely adopted when the provider has to work to get to at them.

Alerts, reminders, and guidelines usually represent the full scope of decision support these days. While forays into artificial intelligence are common in research venues, it has not found wide application among EMRs, perhaps because of physician's distrust, but more often due to technical reasons. This is unfortunate, because truly intelligent systems can markedly reduce the burdens that EMRs place on providers and can support their decisions without intruding upon them.

Patient Education

A second method to support clinical optimization, outside the realm of decision support, is that of patient education materials. The EMR can automate and personalize patient instructions and handouts. For some patients, it is exactly what they need to reinforce what you have told them; other patients promptly recycle the paper. The point of printed education materials is not to comply with mandates, but instead to achieve patient understanding and compliance. Unfortunately, printed education has never been shown to improve compliance. On the other hand, if your providers are spending too much time with the computer, their verbal explanations may be lacking, and this is a nice fall-back.

Optimizing Financial Outcomes

A 2005 analysis of the macroeconomics of EMRs found that for every dollar of benefit the EMR accrues, only 11¢ stays with the physician who pays for the system. The remaining 89¢ flows on downstream, mostly to insurers. I know we are all pleased to continue making money for the insurance industry. After all, it has been costing those poor souls $1.4 million a day(!), squeezed out from between our premiums and our reimbursements, to lobby Congress to avoid the dangers of true healthcare reform legislation.

So you have to stretch your 11¢ as far as you can, to make your EMR pay for itself, and like any budget, it is hard work. Many physicians end up perpetually subsidizing their EMRs without ever realizing it. The break-even point from your initial investment is at minimum a 5-year trajectory. Probably the best financial management model to capture the ongoing return from your EMR is the Net Present Value, which is not difficult to understand, but you would probably prefer to ask your accountant to track it for you.

The trickiest part of securing a true return is recognizing that the cost of the "investment" is nuanced and ongoing. That cost ultimately determines the magnitude of the return. You might have detected some of those (often overlooked) costs in my many comments above, such as the costs of building and maintaining an inventory of templates or the costs of retrieving reportable data. Moreover, the hit on productivity is enormous, and it may be growing. A recent study showed that the average duration of patient visits to primary care has been lengthening, even without the interference of an EMR and despite falling reimbursements. We are already stretching to meet more and more clinical objectives with each encounter; the EMR will make it worse.

The summary is that the total cost of EMR ownership far exceeds the hardware, software, training, and initial customizations, which are the usual pieces included in return on investment (ROI) calculations. Realizing this can help you prior to purchasing the EMR, since that is when you have the most leverage. If your sales representative is promising you improved efficiencies and handsome returns, do two things: (1) ask for real data from a real installation that closely matches your circumstances, and use this to help you model a realistic ROI and (2) get it in writing, and then link the vendor's payment schedule to achieving those goals. Their job is to sell you something, and many of their promises are idealized and unproven. When they promise you the stars, your job is to enlighten them about the emptiness of interstellar space, you crazy Taoist master, you.

True ROI is achieved by reengineering your processes, not by using an EMR per se. There is a vast literature on process reengineering and workflow analysis. It is not a "once and done" analysis of your ideal future state. It should be dynamic and iterative goal setting, changing often.

An important, if subtle, point about process reengineering is that not every step in a process needs to be optimized. In fact, some inefficiencies may need to be designed into your workflow to improve the total efficiency of the system. This observation was formulated by an Israeli physicist, Eliyahu Goldratt, who noticed that any physical system must always have constraints on it, because otherwise it would create a runaway event. Goldratt's Theory of Constraints showed that identifying the constraints on a system was really an exercise in identifying the throttles on the total system's output; and not every throttle needs to be set at maximum to improve your efficiencies.

As a simple illustration, imagine that you are stopped at a traffic light when some hopped-up sports car pulls up beside you. Ahead of you both is a second traffic light, and beyond that, your side of the highway narrows to a single lane. A slow truck is pulling out at the second traffic light, heading toward the single lane, when your light turns green. Either you get ahead of the truck before merging into the single lane, or you are going to suffer miles of being stuck behind the big guy.

Your hot rod friend maximizes speed at every opportunity; it is about as much strategy for passing the truck that his brain can come up with. You, on the other hand, have a more refined sociotechnical symbiosis. You notice that the second light is still red for you, and so you drive more slowly to time it so that you won't have to stop there. Well, you can guess what is going to happen. The hot rod reaches the second light while it is still red, and needs to come to a full stop; meanwhile, you approach the light at less than full speed, it turns green, you calmly pass the stopped hot rod, and then the slow truck as well. By matching your speed to the timing of the light, you have intentionally inserted an inefficiency into one part of your process to maximize the total efficiency.

You will notice the relevance here to clinical practice. We never treat cardiovascular disease without considering a constraint from renal or hepatic function, for example. And our concern about growing bacterial resistance throttles down our use of antibiotics. The health and well-being of our patients is our objective, and to optimize that, we spend every day balancing the constraints from patient and system resources; patient, family and professional preferences; and intersecting disease states. We do not try to maximize every individual thing at once. Instead we try to improve the health of the entire person.

The Theory of Constraints is already a part of your clinical practice, if only intuitively. So when it comes to reengineering your office processes, use that experience to help design a balanced system that optimizes total workflow. It is often repeated that the most expensive item in a practice is the physician's time, so mark that as the global constraint to the flow through your practice and design everything to maximize that. Modify the pace of patient visits and refill requests and telephone messages so that the office staff is catering to the time of the physician.

You might have inefficiencies with your staff's time, granted, but the total workflow will be maximized. In our traffic analogy, the global constraint was the second light, although it would have become the truck if we had not been able to pass it. If something besides physician time becomes your global constraint (such as a procedure room, for example), design your processes to maximize throughput there, even if the physician now has down time.

Notice that process reengineering does not rely upon an EMR to attain its efficiencies. When you insert an EMR into your workflow, you will create entirely new bottlenecks, although you will also introduce new efficiencies. You will not be able to anticipate many of these during the planning phase, which is why optimization is an iterative process of tinkering, trying, observing, and tinkering again. If the physician's time remains your most expensive asset, and the EMR should not have changed that, then every aspect of your EMR customization efforts should be designed to cater to that time. Your staff's jobs get redesigned to compensate for or bypass the EMR's limitations, so the system still maximizes total throughput. At least, that is how to optimize for financial outcomes. What constrains that objective is, of course, optimization of your clinical outcomes, as described above.

There are a number of specific methods for optimizing the financial benefits of your EMR, described below. Before reviewing those, however, a final observation is worth mentioning. We are here considering methods to maximize your financial return using the EMR, which runs counter to the putative point of using an EMR to contain those very costs for the healthcare system. Some questions do not have answers.

Documentation at the Point of Care

If your practice relies on transcription, the potential savings here are substantial and constitute the second most common reason to buy an EMR (the first was improved patient outcomes). You have to appreciate the significant load that eliminating dictation places on a provider. A time motion study found that in a paper-based system, the average physician spends less than 120 seconds recording clinical information about a new patient and only 38 seconds for an established patient visit. The same study found that experienced providers using an EMR took an average of 7.5 minutes on new patients and 4.3 minutes on established patient visits to accomplish the same clinical documentation. Your calculation is as good as mine – that is a nearly 4-fold increase in the time to document a new patient encounter and a whopping 7-fold increase to document the most common type of visit we do. (And that is *not* the 7-fold increase in entering an order.) Yep, you save on transcription, but what was all that about the physician's time being the most expensive asset you've got? Oh yeah.

A big push back can happen here, especially if your providers are uncomfortable with the keyboard. A tip is to break it down: anything less than a paragraph of text is faster with even hunt-and-peck typing, beyond that you might want to try voice recognition (although that comes with its own bottlenecks). Be very careful with cut-and-paste tools and automated text – they are among the most common methods used to expedite documentation, but as mentioned earlier, those notes are being heavily scrutinized.

A point about documentation that is often made by vendors and consultants is that results in other parts of the chart do not have to be included in your note. The reason is that you sign off on having seen those results, so it is redundant to put them back in your note. Maybe that does trim some time off your documentation burden, but doesn't it miss the whole point of the note? In the discussion about managing forms and templates, I tried to emphasize that the reason we sign our notes is, in a sense, to encapsulate the thought to designate the document as a whole unit, an integration of narrative and observations and planning. Again, the black hole model of EMR information is that everything is in there, but none of it comes out in any intelligible form. If the creatinine is relevant to your order to exclude contrast during a CT scan, then do not paste the entire CMP, agreed, but do note the crucial value as a means to document your decision making.

Reduction in Support Staff

This represents the third most common reason for adopting an EMR, specifically, that of reducing operating costs. Managing the paper chart uses a lot of staff time, especially searching for missing charts and reports. The EMR eliminates those constraints, but eliminated positions are often just shifted into new functions, such as scanning, template construction, or network support. Even when the EMR nets a staff reduction, it is often in the form of a fractional position, especially in smaller practices, and that does not do much to reduce expensive employee benefits. Recognize that if staff reduction is one of your highest priorities coming in to the EMR, your final implementation will look very different than if your highest priority was, say, support of your providers.

Attract New Patients

Meeting market and patient expectations is the fourth most common reason for wanting an EMR. For this to be successful, you have to have a marketing strategy. It does not sell itself. Whatever internal chaos your office is experiencing, you want to broadcast a positive, even leading edge, image outside the walls. It is an important training point for those of your staff with direct patient contact. Disgruntlement at the front desk or with your tech will telegraph more to your community than you would like to think. Studies have shown that most patients' impressions about a practice are formed in the first few minutes of walking in the door, well ahead of meeting with you.

Incentives

The fifth most common reason for acquiring an EMR is to engage in some sort of incentive program, and given the recent federal legislation, we are expecting this reason to move up in the rankings. Pay for performance (P4P) programs have been initiated by insurers for some time now. The EMR is supposed to make reporting your measures easier, and it no doubt will do that eventually, but it has not been an especially strong feature to date. An important caveat here was the finding from a recent study that few primary care practices are big enough to actually create statistically meaningful data for performance measures. The practical implication is that our confidence intervals are too broad, and we are really being paid or denied for random variations.

The American Recovery and Reinvestment Act of 2009 included $19 billion of incentives specifically targeted to spur physicians into EMR adoption. These incentives are described in the section known as the Health Information Technology for Economic and Clinical Health Act, or HITECH for short. The incentives take the form of a stepped dispersal over 5 years for a maximum of $44,000, starting in 2011. The total amount of the incentive was derived from the average cost of an EMR in 2004 from across 14 private practices (talk about wide confidence intervals). Practices who do not adopt an EMR during the incentive phase will face reduced reimbursements from CMS thereafter.

The incentives are linked to the definition of "meaningful use" of a "certified" EMR, and CMS proposed its definition for meaningful use on December 30, 2009. The proposed definition has three stages, one progressively building upon the other. Stage 1, starting in 2011, would require physician practices to meet 25 criteria, such as capturing health related information electronically and using decision support tools such as those described above for disease and medication management. Stage 2 would additionally require computerized order entry and electronic interoperability (the ability to transmit and receive orders and test results). Stage 3 would further require reporting on quality and safety indicators, focusing on conditions with high national priority. The third stage would also require patient access to self-management tools.

What constitutes a "certified" EMR is still to be defined by the Office of the National Coordinator for Health Information Technology (ONC). The CMS proposed rule graciously specifies that they will not require certification for which there have not yet been any standards created. Most industry analysts believe that a leading contender for the certifying body is the Certification Commission for Health Information Technology (CCHIT).

A problem with the CMS proposed rule is that it heavily favors practices that already have an EMR and are using it at all. Yes, it is important for those practices, who are likely still subsidizing their own technology, to recoup some of their investment. However, solo practitioners and providers in depressed rural areas would particularly benefit from the incentives but are much less likely to qualify if the final rule remains as proposed. This has the potential to further depress already struggling practices, as the penalty phase of HITECH kicks in, and to further impede access to high quality care by our nation's most vulnerable populations.

A more profound problem with the CMS proposal is that there is no mention of or reward for the process management that is necessary to actually achieve improved patient outcomes and efficiencies in the healthcare system (their stated objectives).

If you have not noticed, I have spent most of these three sections emphasizing that outcome optimization is done with process reengineering. It takes structural changes to create quality improvement, not EMRs per se, and there is no recognition of that fact. The recent experiment in P4P in Great Britain demonstrated clearly that you get *exactly* what you pay for with incentives: paying for 25 criteria, or even 100, will get you exactly those criteria, but no change in outcomes, no shift in mentality toward excellence, and no innovation.

A last problem is that CCHIT is an industry supported group which has been emphasizing tightly integrated products, a stance that heavily favors the existing largest vendors of EMRs. The integration emphasized by the commission so far may stifle some of the innovation necessary to overcome many current problems with EMRs. Recognize that CCHIT has not been chosen by the ONC as of this writing; it just appears to be the likely choice.

A different form of incentive that the EMR might truly assist with is the Clinical and Health Outcomes Initiative in Comparative Effectiveness (CHOICE) program. The Agency for Healthcare Research and Quality (AHRQ) will make $148 million available in 2010 for pragmatic "real patients in real settings" studies and registries, which computers can greatly facilitate.

Enhanced Coding

Realistic industry estimates are that you can achieve around 3–6% of improvement in gross billing when using EMR documentation and coding support. In addition, your entire revenue cycle is sped up with coding and billing from the point of care. On the one hand, physicians have been defensively downcoding for years, worried that their documentation would not survive an audit, and the EMR is simply helping us finally secure our due. On the other hand, Medicare and other insurers are watching very carefully, and they are holding doctors responsible for any overcoding, even when the EMR was being used as intended.

A downside to this optimization is again the shift of burden to providers, many of whom do not feel qualified to correctly code their diagnoses, especially on the fly, or they are completely unaware of how tightly reimbursements can be tied to specific codes. Another downside is that the excessive documentation generated with an EMR to support the higher codes usually amounts to an incoherent jumble of factoids.

Managing the Unpaid Work

How much do you get done in between patients? Wrapping up with whatever still needs to be done for the previous patient, previewing where things are with your next patient, document, grab a bite, help an associate, arrange to pick up the kids, and run the business. And then there is all that unpaid patient care: prescription refills, messages, papers to complete, letters to write, and results to react to. In my office, we move nearly five charts in unpaid work for every chart for a seen patient. All day, every day. Busy does not begin to describe it.

EMRs introduce new possibilities for managing the unpaid work. Prescription refills in particular have the potential to save a lot of time, when issued from an integrated medication list. Messages can also be routed more precisely; decisions can be made quickly when all the information is just a couple clicks away. Here as much as anywhere else, though, it still requires process reengineering, but any reduction in the time spent not getting paid is a positive return.

Information Throughout the Organization

The EMR can be many places at once, and it can supply a single source of truth for your whole system. So if your front staff fixes an address, your tech can correctly send out a reminder. Or when your billing clerk needs to appeal an EOB, the relevant parts of the record can be transmitted right from the desktop. It also allows for true collaboration to occur by having providers and ancillary services each contribute their portions to the whole record. These many small efficiencies can collectively become substantial gains in total workflow.

Less Hassle

This one is definitely not a slam dunk, but EMRs do have features that can reduce hassle. For example, it is a lot less exasperating when you do not have to badger your staff to find the results that the patient came here to review. And just having more complete information at the point of care reduces stress, since no blanks in the record are being guessed at. The value here is hard to quantify, but it can be invaluable, if past inefficiencies were burning out your providers. The happiest providers are always the most productive in terms of both patient numbers and patient satisfaction.

Chapter Conclusion

The January 1910 issue of Scientific American carried an article reporting that automobiles must have reached perfection. The author's conclusion was based on the observation that there had been no substantially new features introduced in the previous 2 years of car shows. But static design does not imply mature technology. With regard to EMRs, we are still running around with buckets of gasoline.

A sociotechnical system is an evolved symbiosis between culture and technology; it takes time, although an occasional asteroid collision helps move it along. Understanding that aspect of the EMR will, I think, help you better navigate both the pitfalls and possibilities of your EMR. Maintenance and optimization are where the rubber meets the road for an EMR. They are complex and intensive efforts. When done with care, they might lead you to Taoist enlightenment, or maybe just a successful EMR implementation and better care of your patients. Your results may vary.

Acknowledgment I would like to acknowledge Sabrina Townsend, RN, Clinical Information Specialist, who gave me very helpful commentary on the early outlines of this chapter. I also want to thank my wife and children, who have borne the brunt of my many late-night meetings and distracted thoughts. Finally, I would like to apologize for the tangle of metaphors, analogies, and wise cracks – it is just how I explain things.

References

1. Han YY, Carcillo JA, Venkataraman ST, et al. Unexpected increased mortality after imple-mentation of a commercially sold computerized physician order entry system. *Pediatrics*. 2005;116(6):1506–1512.
2. Chin T. Doctors pull the plug on paperless system. *Am Med News*. 2003;Feb 17:1,4.

Suggested Reading

The following readings are easy to get through and very focused, for the most part. The exceptions are Goldratt's novel, which is a fast read, although you will need to pay attention to notice what he is saying, and the CMS proposed rule, which is 550 pages, although the link provided is a one-page summary. These readings by no means constitute a complete reference for all the aspects involved in EMR maintenance and optimization, but they may help reinforce key concepts or introduce you to the larger literature basis for this section.

Regarding Low EMR Adoption Rates, High Resistance Levels, and High Failure Rates

DesRoches CM, Campbell EG, Rao SR, et al. Electronic health records in ambulatory care – A national survey of physicians. *N Engl J Med*. 2008;359:50–60.
Ford EW, Menachemi N, Petersona LT, Huerta TR. Resistance is futile: But it is slowing the pace of EHR adoption nonetheless. *J Am Med Inform Assoc*. 2009;16:274–281.
Littlejohns P, Wyatt JC, Garvican L. Evaluating computerised health information systems: Hard lessons still to be learnt. *BMJ*. 2003;326:860–863.

Regarding Your Mindset – the Fuzzy Trace Theory and Sociotechnical Systems

Wilkinson TM. Medical reasoning and the failure of electronic medical record systems in the United States. *Int J Clin Pract*. 2010;64(7):839–842.
Reyna VF. A theory of medical decision making and health: Fuzzy trace theory. *Med Decis Making*. 2008;28(6):850–865.

Wears RL, Berg M. Computer technology and clinical work: Still waiting for Godot. *JAMA*. 2005;293(10):1261–1263.

Regarding EULAs

Silverstein S. Health care information technology, hospital responsibilities, and Joint Commission standards. *JAMA*. 2009;302(4):382–383.

Regarding the Persistence of Paper with Mature EMR Systems

Saleem JJ, Russ AL, Justice CF, Hagg H, Ebright PR, Woodbridge PA, Doebbeling BN. Exploring the persistence of paper with the electronic health record. *Int J Med Inform*. 2009;78:618–628.

Regarding the Macroeconomics of EMRs

Bates DW. Physicians and ambulatory electronic health records. *Health Aff (Millwood)*. 2005;24(5):1181–1189.

Regarding the Theory of Constraints

Goldratt, EM, Cox J. *The Goal: A Process of Ongoing Improvement, 3e*. Croton-on-Hudson, NY: North River Press; 2004.

Regarding the $44,000 Stimulus and P4P

Miller RH, West C, Brown TM, Sim I, Ganchoff C. The value of electronic health records in solo or small group practices. *Health Aff (Millwood)*. 2005;24(5)1127–1137.

Campbell SM, Reeves D, Kontopantelis E, Sibbald B, Roland M. Effects of pay for performance on the quality of primary care in England. *N Engl J Med*. 2009;361:368–378.

CMS proposed definition of "meaningful use": http://www.cms.hhs.gov/apps/media/press/factsheet.asp?Counter=3564

Chapter 7
A View from the Top: Reflections of Leaders in the Electronic Health Record Industry

Neil S. Skolnik

> *The computer is a logic machine, and that is its strength – but also its limitation. The important events on the outside cannot be reported in the kind of form a computer could possibly handle. Man, however, while not particularly logical is perceptive – and that is his strength.*
> – Peter Drucker, the Effective Executive

Abstract This chapter is comprised of responses from chief executive officers and chief medical officers of some of the major EHR vendors addressing two questions – what should clinicians be looking for now as they consider purchasing an EHR for their practice and where they feel the industry is going, that is to say what changes will we be seeing over the next 5 years of which the practicing physician should be aware. The expectation was that their thoughts would be interesting, but fairly consistent, in their positive outlook of the EHR industry and the promises of what EHRs might do for patient care. After all, they are the leaders in a industry which will change the way that health care is delivered more than any other single invention or discovery of this generation. Instead, what you will see in this chapter is that while their views are positive about the potential for EHRs to improve care, their views are anything but consistent as they speak honestly of the potential promises and pitfalls facing both the industry and the individual practitioners in choosing and implementing EHRs.

Keywords Experiences · Opinions · CEO · Trust · Selection · Safety · Costs · Future · Function · Technology · Affordability · Innovation · Perspective

N.S. Skolnik (✉)
Family Medicine Residency Program, Abington Memorial Hospital and Professor of Family and Community Medicine, Temple University School of Medicine, Philadelphia, PA, USA
e-mail: nskolnik@comcast.net

N.S. Skolnik (ed.), *Electronic Medical Records*, Current Clinical Practice,
DOI 10.1007/978-1-60761-606-1_7, © Springer Science+Business Media, LLC 2011

In the second chapter we looked at the experiences and opinions of primary care physicians who had implemented EHRs in their offices. Their experience varied enormously. For almost all the physicians, introducing an EHR to their practice created both anticipated and unanticipated challenges and the journey to successful implementation, when successful implementation occurred, was usually filled with fits and starts. For some physicians having an EHR has allowed them to better organize their practice, more efficiently find charts, and access information both in and out of their office. For other physicians, bringing an EHR into their office was a nightmare that decreased clinical productivity and impeded patient care without any significant improvement in the quality of care.

My expectation in asking chief executive officers and chief medical officers of some of the major EHR vendors to reflect on what was important to them was that their thoughts would be interesting, but fairly consistent, in their positive outlook of the EHR industry and the promises of what EHRs might do for patient care. After all, they are the leaders in a industry which will change the way that health care is delivered more than any other single invention or discovery of this generation. Instead, what you will see is that while their views are certainly positive about the potential for EHRs to improve care, their views are anything but consistent and they speak honestly of the potential promises and pitfalls facing both the industry and the individual practitioners in choosing and implementing EHRs. All these individuals are extremely busy, so I thank all of them for giving generously of their time and efforts in contributing to this chapter.

The authors where essentially asked to address two questions – what should clinicians be looking for now as they consider purchasing an EHR for their practice, and where is the industry going, that is to say what changes will we be seeing over the next 5 years of which the practicing physician should be aware. How they chose to organize the essay was up to the individual author. The task of writing an essay to these questions was meant to provide an opportunity for these leaders to think about and describe their perspective on the future of the industry as well as what is currently important to patients and providers. The request emphasized that they should try to give information that would be helpful to primary care physicians as they choose, implement, and optimize an EHR in their office. To be fair, the essays are published in the order in which they were submitted back after requests for the essay where sent.

What You Don't Know CAN Hurt You

David L. Winn

David L. Winn, M.D., FAAFP is founder, chair and lead developer on e-MDs next generation web native EHR.

Who Can You Trust to Help in the EHR Selection Process?

The problem with EHRs is there is no one trustworthy source that a physician can rely on to help in the selection process. Vendor user forums are good for discussing the pros and cons of the vendor's EMR, but do not provide any useful comparative information. Public forums suffer from "trolls" with their own bias and hidden agendas. There are many good consultants, but just as many bad ones who recommend a product based on the complexity of the installation and their comparably higher consulting fees (sad, but very true). Perhaps the best overall source for vendor selection is your specialty's web site. Several different academies including the AAFP, ACP, AAN, and ACP have sections devoted to physician satisfaction with their EHR choice. The academies are largely protected from manipulation by vendors. Word of mouth can also be helpful, although some practices are compensated for favorable review, so vendor-offered references may be less objective.

What Else Is Important in the EHR Selection Process?

Do not allow your staff to pick the EHR. This may be the most important take home message from this book! What you ask?..... this is sacrilege. Every other self help guide says get staff involved in the selection process early. Yes and no. Staff and physicians have different needs and wants. Not all EHRs are equally good at charting as they are in front office functions. Slick scheduling and front office workflow functions will be very appealing to staff – where they spend the majority of their time in the application. Physicians, on the other hand, spend the majority of their time in the Chart where HPI, diagnosis, orders, and e-prescribing (CPOE) must be fast and efficient. Many EHR installations have failed because the physicians delegated the important task of the EHR selection to the CFO, office manager, or staff without understanding the full impact of a second rate charting component on usability and speed of documentation.

Think about this. If one EHR excels at charting – perhaps improving a physician's efficiency/productivity by 5%, while at the same time, suffering from a less elegant front office interface – let us presume degrading the efficiency of the non-clinical staff by 5 or even 10%, which EHR is the better choice? The calculation is pretty straight forward. A physician's time is worth a minimum of $300–$400 per hour; some specialists double or triple this. The front office staff are a cost center averaging around 3 FTEs per physician at an hourly rate of $15–$20/hour.

That said, it is important to explain the rationale behind your decision making to your staff and it is critical to involve them at every level for a successful implementation. If you ultimately select the best "Charting" solution rather than the best "front office" solution, your staff, at first, may be a bit resentful. If the better charting solution improves practice income as advertised, why not reward loyal staff who contributed to a successful roll out with some form of profit sharing?

Finally, beware of "eye candy" and the "demo dolly." Eye candy is software that is exceptionally pleasing to the eye. A great deal of thought has gone into making the user facing interface appealing and in the hands of an expert "demo dolly", the software demo appears almost magical in how well it works. These are superficial visual treats and in real world scenarios these systems often break down in usability, form, and function. A scripted demo is almost worthless. How well the EHR works in the fast paced, real world clinical "battlefield" is what really counts.

Is Considering the Safety of the EHR Really an Issue? Are not They All Equally Safe?

Unfortunately no. Senator Grassley sent a letter on October 16, 2009 to 10 major EHR vendors expressing concern over software errors that might lead to patient injury or death. He missed a few! What these companies all have in common is the fierce, investor driven competition to include as many features as possible, as fast as possible. Without adequate testing, supervision, or perhaps even regard for patient safety, these EHRs are being perpetrated on unsuspecting public and unsuspecting physicians. These companies do have one thing in common. They are exceptionally good at sales and marketing. Take note that no physician led EHR company has EVER had a patient safety complaint. Why is that? Remember from medical school the axiom *"**Primum non nocere**"?* It means first, do no harm. The single most important point that we drive home to our developers and testers is we will not allow our product into production with any error that might compromise patient safety. Period. If somehow an error is missed that might somehow jeopardize patient safety (this happened just once to e-MDs with a patient record duplication bug), we immediately "stop the presses" and put all hands on solving the problem above all else. One major, well known ambulatory vendor has had a medication prescribing error of one form or another since 2005 and it continues to re-emerge – as recently as October 2009! This is a well known problem and they cannot or will not spend the effort to resolve it! The physicians who use the product are not happy about it and complain loudly on their user forum, yet the problems persist. The same vendor also has a gaping privacy/security problem that has been described on the same user forum. I can only speculate that physicians continue to use this product because of the significant investment they have made in the product and the fear that coming forward might damage the ongoing viability of their vendor.

What Are the Hidden Costs?

These are often hard to quantify and vendors are loath to bring it up, but consider the costs after the sale. If a vendor's application requires a third party to customize it, typically billing out at a rate of $100–$150 per hour, you can quickly run up large, unanticipated fees. How easy is the application to use? A product that does everything, only does everything if you can figure out how to "unlock" the feature. Some highly rated (not the same as highly regarded) products, based on an extensive checklist of features, have a very high failure rate due to their enormous complexity. If a complex EHR slows you down for the first 6 months (not uncommon), the real cost may be MUCH higher than the original quoted price. If physician productivity is negatively impacted by 25% for 6 months (the norm rather than the exception), the additional cost of the application to the average primary care physician can approach $50,000!

Predicting the Future

As cloud computing becomes more pervasive and accepted, EHRs will slowly migrate away from the local area network to centralized, hosted solutions on remote servers. The only thing holding this back has been an inconsistent internet backbone and a few well publicized security breaches. The Apple iPad, despite its limitations (and choice of name), is an excellent, inexpensive platform for the mobile, browser based EHR. If it is dropped or stolen there is no compromise of data – just grab another one off the desk. The enormous complexity and "bloat" of today's apps will give way to lean, Google like simplicity and ease of use. The power will be there, but cognitive engineering will allow comparable form and function to stay hidden until needed. Frequently needed functions will "append" to the toolbar as the system monitors each user for his or her individual preferences and usage patterns. Interoperability, that is, the ability of computers to share, comprehend, and perform operations on medical information, will take another 10 years to fully develop as established vendors try desperately to protect their proprietary systems AND obscene profits. Software as a service – combining software with such activities as billing optimization, quality reporting and even disease management will slowly erode the strangle hold that many large vendors have today on the health information technology space. Finally, doctors will discover, perhaps painfully, that they MUST be in control of their patient's data. Saving a few dollars up front by turning over control to hospitals or mega corporations will ultimately extract a heavy price in continued erosion of physician autonomy and decision making.

The EHR will someday prove to be the physician's twenty-first century equivalent to penicillin in the fight to save lives and improve care, but the fight will be long and bloody with physician and patient casualties along the way. For those who persevere, who do the research and filter out the sales/marketing hype to pick a good EHR, the rewards will be huge for physician and patient alike. Picking the wrong EHR, however, will be an expensive and morale destroying mistake from which some physicians will likely never recover. The risks are great, but the reward is greater.

Going, Going, There: How Current EHR Initiatives Can Help Shape Buying Decisions

Sarah Corley, MD, Chief Medical Officer, NextGen Healthcare

Sarah Corley is the Chief Medical Officer for NextGen Healthcare Information Systems, an Electronic Health Record (EHR) vendor. She also practices part time as a primary care Internist in the metropolitan Washington, DC area. She attended medical school and completed her Internal Medicine residency at the University of Virginia where she first was exposed to health information technology (HIT). She received post-graduate training in Medical Informatics at OHSU. She practiced primary care Internal Medicine for 15 years with gradually increasing involvement in informatics before moving full time into Health Informatics. She has used EHRs in her practice since 1994. She served a 4-year term as Governor of the Virginia Chapter of the American College of Physicians (ACP) and a 6-year term on their National Medical Informatics Subcommittee. She has participated on a number of national panels on the topic of health information technology in clinical practice. She currently serves as a Commissioner for the Certification Commission for Healthcare Information Technology. She represents the ACP on the Physicians EHR Coalition. She served on a number of workgroups and expert panels on an assortment of HIT topics. Her research interest lies in using EHRs to improve quality in medical practices.

The need to improve the quality of care while lowering its cost is at the root of every major initiative in healthcare today. While new models of care are evolving to meet this need, new technology applications are being developed simultaneously to make these models viable. The EHR is both the means and the end of these revolutionary processes.

An EHR's raison d'être is to collect and share data important for the treatment of patients. This seemingly simple function, however, rests on complex, multifaceted relationships that seek to balance caregivers' needs against information systems' capabilities. Driven forward by federal government mandates, the next several years promise to bring issues of EHR standardization, usability, and interoperability to the forefront of practicing physicians' collective awareness.

EHR Development: Where It Is Going, and Why

While change is constant in healthcare – and exponential in technology – three EHR developmental imperatives are emerging in response to industry trends, as well as existing and imminent federal requirements:

1. **Interoperability**. Standardization – the prerequisite for sharing records between and among IT systems – has been an important, though hard to achieve, goal of EHR development since 1991, when the Institute of Medicine's report, *The Computer-based Patient Record: An Essential Technology for Health Care*, introduced the idea of "an electronic patient record ... specifically designed to support users through availability of complete and accurate data, alerts, reminders, clinical decision support systems, links to medical knowledge and other aids." (1) Since that time, several organizations have worked to further

the development of standards, with some success as evidenced by standardization of lab results, medication names, allergies, and demographic data. Other data elements, such as physician progress notes that require multiple concepts to express, are proving more problematic. The challenge is ensuring interoperability for public health reporting and research without hindering or further complicating the physician "conversation." Meeting this challenge demands ongoing, industry-level standards development.

2. **Usability**. As federal mandates increase quality and reporting requirements, EHR solutions must evolve to help rather than hinder physicians' efforts to meet them. For example, an EHR that requires numerous "clicks" to order a single medication is not going to streamline a physician's workflow. The problem is finding ways to objectively measure something as seemingly subjective as usability.

   However, the issue is now on the federal radar and fast becoming a must-have for EHR products. Certification organizations increasingly are looking for ways to measure and mandate usability of EHR products, from the National Institute of Standards and Technology's (NIST) search for sources "to fully develop and execute a project to create a usability framework for health information technology (HIT) systems" (2) to the Certified Commission for Healthcare Information Systems' (CCHIT) 2011 Usability Testing Guide for Comprehensive Ambulatory EHRs.

3. **Care coordination**. Despite spending one sixth of our entire gross domestic product on healthcare, the US falls far short of being the healthiest society in the world. One reason is that we spend the vast majority of our resources treating the symptoms rather than the causes of disease. Care coordination across all elements of the complex healthcare system (e.g., subspecialty care, hospitals, home health agencies, nursing homes, etc.) and the patient's community is essential to creating a shift from treatment to prevention – and EHRs are essential to care coordination. In addition, care coordination is a key characteristic of the Patient-Centered Medical Home (PCMC), an emerging care concept based on evidence, driven by data, focused on health and wellness, and centered on the needs of the patient.

These three imperatives – interoperability, usability and care coordination – are driving EHR development. As such, they also are key considerations in the selection of an EHR solution.

Functional Matters: Choosing an EHR Solution

The 2009 American Recovery and Reinvestment Act's (ARRA) HITECH Act may have brought EHRs to the forefront of healthcare discussion, but it did not alter their primary function – improving the quality of care. To ensure this result, physicians should look for the following in an EHR product:

- Certification:Certification assures that a product has met core criteria considered essential by a broad range of stakeholders, which is key to maximizing the system's value. One-time certification is not enough; annual certification evidences the continual development necessary for the product's ongoing viability.

  The sole organization designated by Health and Human Services (HHS) since 2006, CCHIT is the industry's leading EHR certification body and the de facto standard for usability and other criteria. However, with the advent of ARRA and the resulting need to preclude any conflict of interest, HHS now will oversee multiple certification organizations. The Office of the National Coordinator (ONC) for Health Information Technology is developing its own certification criteria with NIST, which will assess conformity and accredit certification bodies. Still, those that now possess CCHIT usability ratings and certification have positioned themselves in the forefront of the certification process.
- Structured data: Structured data resides in fixed fields within a record or file. These discrete data fields (e.g., blood pressure, body mass index, and height/weight) establish the predetermined data types and understood relationships necessary for efficient quality reporting. Since 2008, the Centers for Medicare & Medicaid Services (CMS) has allowed reporting of quality measures data to a qualified registry. As early as this year, CMS could begin accepting direct EHR-based quality reporting. As early as 2012, CMS could mandate it. EHRs built on unstructured data (as is found in many transcription/dictation systems) will not support compliance.
- Meaningful use guarantees: Incentives should not be the sole reason why physicians deploy EHRs, but the ability to secure incentives must not be overlooked. EHR vendors with a commitment to – and a plan for – meeting meaningful use criteria as they are established will offer guarantees to that effect.
- Clinical decision support: Evidence-based practice is the inevitable future of healthcare. EHRs with clinical prompts and reminders support best practice and systemize the use of evidence at the point of care.
- Support for coordinated care: Increasingly, EHRs will serve as the foundation for data registries, health information exchange, and other means to assure patients get the indicated care when and where they need and want it, and in a culturally and linguistically appropriate manner. Expanded patient data access – via secure communication portals, for instance – also will require more robust data controls to ensure secure data exchange. However, it will enable patient-centric care through greater patient involvement.

Healthcare is a dynamic industry, driven by the needs – changing and continuous – of its stakeholders. Developing, choosing, and deploying EHRs will continue to challenge. Keeping standardization, usability, and interoperability as the prime focus of all development and purchase decisions ultimately will smooth the path for everyone.

1. The Computer-Based Patient Record: An Essential Technology for Health Care Committee on Improving the Patient Record, Division of Health Care

Services, Institute of Medicine Richard S. Dick, Elaine B. Steen; eds. 190 pages. Washington, D.C.: National Academy Press; 1991.
2. National Institute of Standards and Technology. Health Information Technology Usability Framework. Federal Business Opportunity. Solicitation Number: AMD-10-SS39 Web. https://www.fbo.gov/index?s=opportunity&mode=form&id=9a64d99691f54a9948ca65442c5fe6a7&tab=core&_cview=0

Back to the Future: Using EHRs to Make the Practice of Medicine All that It Once Was...and More

John H. Hammergren, Chairman and Chief Executive Officer of McKesson Corporation

John H. Hammergren is Chairman, President, and Chief Executive Officer of McKesson Corporation. He has been a director of McKesson since 1999 and was elected President and CEO in 2001 and Chairman in 2002. Under Hammergren's leadership, McKesson has emerged as the leading provider of supply, information, and care management solutions designed to reduce the cost and improve the quality of healthcare. During his tenure, the company has more than doubled revenues to $106B and advanced to number 15 on the Fortune 500.

Since 2009, Hammergren has been Chairman of the Healthcare Leadership Council, a coalition of chief executives of leading health care organizations. He is also a member of the Hewlett Packard board of directors, the Business Council, and the Business Roundtable. Hammergren earned a BA in business administration from the University of Minnesota and an MBA from Xavier University.

Practicing medicine today is not what it used to be – much to the chagrin of many great physicians. Indeed, doctors are struggling with a long list of burdens that have taken some of the luster off of the medical profession.

A substantial decline in real income. Spiraling malpractice insurance costs. The need to care for an aging population with more complex care requirements. A shrinking clinical workforce. The realization that in most cases, reimbursement is still tied to the quantity of care delivered, not to patient wellness and outcomes. These are just a few of the challenges that are making it difficult for physicians to run effective practices – and to take care of their own financial well-being.

Add to the mix the fact that physicians deliver the best recommended care to their patients only about 55% of the time – in an era when consumers are actually becoming more demanding – and it is easy to see why frustration runs rampant.

It is not surprising then that many physicians look back with nostalgia and perhaps more than a touch of envy at the past, when medicine was practiced in a Dr. Marcus Welby-like fashion. Indeed, physicians long for the days when they could form close personal bonds with their patients and have a true impact on the quality of their patients' lives versus rushing through one 15-minute appointment after the next day in and day out.

As a result, they are apt to wonder: "Will the practice of medicine ever be as satisfying and enriching as it once was?" Although most probably assume those days are long lost, from my perspective as CEO of the largest healthcare services and information technology companies in the country, I believe that the practice of medicine can be all that it once was – and more.

My vision is for a healthcare system where technology and innovation lead to better health for all Americans. Where the extended care team – doctors, nurses, pharmacists and others – can coordinate care across settings. And where costs are lower and care is safer. It is not going to be easy, but I think we are on the precipice of what could truly evolve into a new, greatly improved era of medicine.

A New Focus

To get there, however, we need to cast our industry in a new light. More specifically, we must remove all of the moral, political, and social rhetoric inherent in the current healthcare reform debate and look at the healthcare crisis for what it is: A business problem.

By doing so, it becomes much easier to do what business people do best: Identify challenges and implement solutions. For instance, it becomes readily apparent that the industry is stumbling due to outdated information technology; poor application of basic market economics principles; overall inefficiency in terms of work flow, care delivery and the spreading of best practices; a lack of transparency around quality and costs; and blocked access to making informed consumer choices.

Clearly, part of the answer to these problems includes not only the acceptance but the enthusiastic adoption of technology. For physicians in particular, technology can become a critical enabler of improved business, operational, and clinical performance.

Among the many technologies available to support physician practices, EHRs offer some of the broadest and most compelling benefits. These systems can help physician practices reduce errors, paperwork, and inefficiencies. As a matter of fact, EHRs have been proven to enhance staff productivity, making it possible for medical groups to do more with less, improve revenue through more accurate clinical coding, and decrease costs by reducing transcription expenses.

Such improvements can help physicians get on track financially and recoup the time they need to do what matters most – caring for patients. Imagine that physicians can spend less time chasing down charts and payments and more time engaging with their patients and concentrating on the practice of medicine.

Great Expectations

The core productivity benefits of EHRs, however, are only the start. EHRs will help clinicians provide better care than they ever dreamed possible. By choosing to use EHRs that integrate with other systems, provide access to clinical knowledge, and offer advanced patient communication functionality, physicians can practice medicine on a higher plane than ever before.

Not only will physicians have the time to truly engage with patients – just as the fictional Dr. Welby did – but they will also be empowered to deliver best practice, evidence-based care in each and every patient encounter. That's something even the most effective clipboard-toting doctors could never do.

For example, clinical decision support can help physicians leverage the latest research and best practices on a day-to-day basis. Consider the following: We already know a lot about heart disease, but unfortunately physicians do not always leverage this knowledge at the point of care. Under our current system, physicians are unable to turn proven remedies into everyday protocols. Half of the people who need heart attack prevention treatment are not treated, and the remaining half are treated inadequately. By pushing clinical support to physicians, our healthcare system can reduce the impact of heart attacks and save some 500,000 lives each year.

Integrating with other systems and sharing information will make an even greater impact. Physician practices can use EHRs to securely exchange information with other practices, patients, hospitals and payors, As physicians begin to share performance data, consumers can make more informed decisions, and physicians can objectively analyze how well they are serving patients and make targeted improvements.

Fortunately, one of the most significant barriers to technology adoption, funding, has now been largely addressed. With the American Recovery and Reinvestment Act providing incentives for the adoption of EHRs and many healthcare IT companies offering financing programs to cover the start-up costs, physicians can overcome that initial hurdle.

With these new incentives and funding mechanisms in place, I believe we are ready to usher forth a revolution in healthcare. By adopting a business orientation and leveraging technology, physicians will be able to help move the healthcare industry forward and create an environment that ensures:

- Everyone gets the care they need, when they need it.
- Patients are positioned at the center of their own care decisions, empowered to make informed choices based on quality, convenience. and costs.
- Care providers coordinate referrals, tests, appointments, treatments, follow-up, and payments seamlessly.
- Errors, waste, and long waits are eliminated.
- Innovations in diagnosis, treatment, and delivery are consistently being made and quickly spread, creating new standards of best practice that benefit everyone.

With EHRs and other healthcare information technology, the high-tech productivity and quality boom experienced by other industries is finally catching up to healthcare, making a fully digital and integrated system possible for the first time. The future has never looked brighter, and with the rapid advancement of EHRs, the future is happening now.

Picking the Right EHR: A Few Simple Steps to Find a Usable and Affordable System

Jonathan Bertman, MD, FAAFP

Dr. Bertman is Clinical Assistant Professor of Family Medicine at the Warren Alpert Medical School at Brown University and is the Physician Editor-in-Chief of MDNG / MD Net Guide. He is the founder and president of AmazingCharts.com, a leading developer of EHR software and AfraidToAsk.com, a consumer health-information website. He has a private practice in Hope Valley, Rhode Island.

As a Family Physician and the president of Amazing Charts, an EHR company that focuses on small practices like my own, I get to see the EHR industry from both a physician and a vendor perspective. One would like to believe that both sides work as partners to promote successful EHR adoptions where everybody ends up satisfied. Unfortunately, this is not the case, and it turns out that it is the unwary physician that all too often gets the short end of the stick.

Proof of this is the astounding percentage of practices that have paid thousands for an EHR only to have it sit, under-utilized, or unused, on their computers. In fact, it is estimated that more than 1/3 of all attempted EHR implementations fail. And this alarming number is expected to increase substantially as the less technologically savvy among us are pressured by the government and third-party payers to adopt health technology.

But using some simple common sense, which is surprisingly overlooked by many otherwise quite intelligent physicians, will ensure that you will nott experience the buyer's remorse that a good number of your colleagues will, or already are, experiencing. Simply asking yourself two simple questions will not only save you hours upon hours of frustration, it will also save you thousands upon thousands of dollars.

- Is the system proven to be USABLE?
- Is the system truly AFFORDABLE?

As an overworked physician in a practice where reimbursements are low and money is always tight, it is obvious that these two points are all that really matter. Finding the answers to these common sense questions is relatively easy, and focusing on these two points while ignoring all the other marketing hype and vendor promises, will ensure you do not end up in the group of physicians who have already made a time-consuming and costly mistake.

Vendors are adept at demonstrating their software to prospective buyers, and as they walk through the software, highlighting cool features and exciting abilities, it is easy to forget that most of the "bells whistles" shown do not actually improve the speed with which a note can be written. In fact, many of these features actually hamper the ability to quickly document a note. A common example of this is the robust template technologies that many vendors proudly demonstrate. At first glance, most physicians are impressed with the ability of an EHR to generate sentences from what appears to be just a few clicks.

In reality, each mouse-click, menu selection, and sub-menu and pop-up window navigation takes a couple of seconds or more, and these momentary lags quickly add up. Add to that the time it takes to find the correct choice from within a list of items, and documenting a simple finding suddenly takes more time than it would to dictate or hand-write the information.

It is only recently, as more physicians have learned the hard way that dozens to hundreds of clicks to document a brief visit just is not practical, that their collective frustration has led to user-satisfaction surveys and closer analysis of what makes an EHR usable. Reviewing this actual user experience before choosing an EHR is imperative. Excluding vendors that do not have a high user rating, or those without enough active clients to be included in these studies, is a practical first step at weeding out the EHRs that have not been proven to be usable in a live practice setting. One interesting finding of these user-satisfaction studies is that, more often than not, the more expensive an EHR, the less usable its users rate it.

In addition to comparing EHR systems in terms of usability, finding those that are truly affordable is also obvious yet frequently ignored. One issue is that that a number of systems have been designed to require expensive servers, complicated networking, and the IT personnel to support these. For the sake of brevity, we will ignore these differences and focus solely on the cost of the software and any required modules (e.g., e-prescribing, E&M coding, training, etc.). As one looks at EHR pricing, it quickly becomes apparent that there is a huge variation, from free open source programs to those costing $40,000 per physician or more.

As demonstrated by user-satisfaction surveys, EHR pricing is unrelated to usability – in fact the relationship appears to be more inversely proportionate. Similarly, pricing is not based on certification status, as many lower-priced systems have the same certification level as higher-priced systems. In fact, there are no tangible factors to explain why one program costs $1000 while a second costs $10,000 and a third costs $40,000. For the vast majority of products that consumers purchase, price tends to be a function of the underlying cost of production and overall quality; EHR pricing is based on neither.

Personally, I believe that EHR pricing is artificially elevated due to the young age of this industry combined with government and third-party payers pressure and incentives to adopt health technology before there is an obvious incentive for the practicing physician. In fact, since the government is promising up to $44,000 in payments to physicians who use a certified EHR in a meaningful way, most software companies will continue to charge these prices until such money is no longer available. At that time, however, the price of EHRs will drop precipitously as actual competition becomes the driving force and vendors must provide better solutions at a lower cost, or lose out to their competitors.

In the meantime, EHR vendors have various means of obscuring their true cost. Some will not even provide a price unless you agree to allow them to come and demonstrate their system. For those that provide more transparent pricing, many will hide "extras" until such time as you actually ask – and that is usually after a prospective buyer has already spent a lot of time and energy on the system. For example, there are vendors that quote a software price, and then tell you later that it costs three times that amount for the EHR training they mandate. Many vendors charge fees not quoted in their software cost for "additional functionality" that is required to practice medicine, such as e-Prescribing, E&M Coding, laboratory interfaces, etc. Another technique used to make comparing actual pricing difficult is to quote a monthly lease price as is done for most ASP-type products. Finding a way to compare product cost is essential to making an informed decision and avoid overpaying for software that may be difficult to use.

Here are a few steps to increase the odds that you will end up satisfied with your EHR choice:

1. Start by selecting only EHR vendors that have high user-satisfaction ratings.
2. Of these, find those that provide transparent pricing on their website. Be sure to ask about features that may not be included, but are obviously required, such as e-Prescribing or additional charges for training. Exclude vendors that seem to hide these costs until you specifically ask: if they are acting unethically now, do you really want to enter a long-term relationship with them?
3. Along this line, a good litmus test of a vendor's ethics is how they market the HITECH stimulus money. Yes, officially each physician can get up to $44,000 over 5 years for adopting a certified EHR in a meaningful way. Unfortunately, the legislation actually says that physicians will be provided up to 75% of their individual Medicare collections up to a maximum of $44,000. Many of us generate significantly less in Medicare payments and are thus only eligible to receive up to 75% of the amount we generate. A company that implies that choosing their software will provide the physician up to 44 K and thus offset their price is being deceptive – and is one I would advise you to avoid.
4. Of the vendors that are left, select the vendors who provide a free trial or full money-back guarantee, so you can prove that their software is actually usable in your practice. Exclude vendors that are not confident enough in their software to provide this obvious "try before you buy" guarantee. Similarly, many companies are promising incentive money or they will give you your money back. Again, read the fine-print. Some of the more unethical companies will state the money they will give you back is much less than the implied full price you have paid.
5. Finally, since it is quite likely that vendor pricing will decrease once EHR adoption incentives and stimulus monies dry up, get the vendor to guarantee in writing that if they lower their price in the future, they will refund back to you the difference. Why should you be penalized for purchasing their software now?

In summary, using the key points of usability and affordability peppered with a bit of common sense, you can protect yourself and your money, while ensuring you will end up in the group who love their EHR, and not in the ever-growing list of physicians who picked the wrong EHR.

Today's EHR Choice Is Critical to a Physician Practice's Future Success

Glen Tullman

Glen Tullman is chief executive officer of Chicago-based Allscripts (NASDAQ: MDRX), the leading provider of clinical software, connectivity and information solutions that physicians use to improve healthcare. He joined the company in August 1997 as CEO to lead the Company's transition into the Healthcare Information Sector.

Physicians who want to acquire an EHR today have a lot to consider. Most obviously, they need to be certain that the EHR they select will enable them to demonstrate meaningful use so they can qualify for the government incentives offered under the American Recovery and Reinvestment Act (ARRA), both in 2011 and afterward. Beyond that, physicians have to prepare for a future in which "pay for quality" is going to become an increasingly important part of Medicare reimbursement (and private insurance payments, too, if history is any guide). Population health management and improved care coordination, based on robust electronic connectivity among providers, will also be required. And, to facilitate greater patient engagement in their own care, physician practices will need to provide patients online access to their own medical records.

Besides meeting these objectives, the EHR must be designed to meet the unique requirements of the physician practice, regardless of its size and specialty. It should be a physician-developed and tested product – because software developers do not understand a physician's everyday challenges – and one that is easy to implement and use in everyday practice. The EHR should enable its users to both improve the quality of care they provide and the reporting on that care, and it should include a patient portal that enables physicians to upload key portions of a patient's record for secure online access. Finally, and perhaps most importantly, the EHR must be able to connect online with key healthcare stakeholders including not only patients but other providers, payers, pharmacies, labs, and the EHRs of other vendors. Connectivity is critical as a basic requirement of the meaningful use criteria, but also to optimize care coordination.

Few characteristics are more important in an EHR provider than a long track record of success. This is especially so today, because many smaller EHR vendors are expected to fall by the wayside as the meaningful use requirements become more challenging. Physicians will need to ensure that the vendor or partner they select has the "staying power" and the resources to invest in software that will not only satisfy today's requirements but, equally important, tomorrow's desires. The greatest risk physicians face is not that the EHR they select turns out to lack a particular feature or function. As is common across the software industry, the top competitors will continue to leapfrog each other and "imitate" new ideas from competitors. The far greater risk is buying from a vendor that goes out of business, forcing physicians not only to start over but to transfer all of their patient data to a new EHR – an arduous and expensive process. For that reason, it is advisable not to choose a vendor, but to choose a long-term business partner you like.

A key part of the selection process is to examine how other groups of the same size and specialty have performed on a particular EHR product. Have they been able to use it to improve the quality of care and achieve a return on investment? If they have, then similar practices should be able to repeat their results using the same technology.

Product Support and Innovation

As the ARRA incentives lead more physicians to search for an EHR, innovation will become a key differentiator, as it has in other industries. The winners will be companies with the size and development resources to create unique physician-focused and patient-focused innovations that deliver higher quality patient care, reduce dangerous drug interactions, and take out costs.

A perfect example of this kind of innovation is illustrated by the advances being made in mobile healthcare IT applications that enhance the usefulness of EHRs, particularly when physicians are on call. Anytime, anywhere access to and control of their EHR from an iPhone, BlackBerry or Windows Mobiles and other smart phones will be important. This enables physicians to safely make critical medical decisions even when they are away from the office, with all relevant information available on the one device they keep closest – their phone. Capabilities can include quick access to real-time patient summary information such as problem lists and medications; the ability to electronically transmit a copy of the patient's record to the nearest hospital emergency room, including notes dictated directly into the iPhone; ePrescribing to the patient's regular pharmacy; and real-time access to all the information a physician needs to make decisions, including medical history, lab results, and medications.

Other innovations include computer kiosks that utilize biometric authentication technology. These devices speed patient check-in, more easily collect vital demographic information such as changes in insurance coverage, and enable patients to charge their co-payments and get alerts about overdue health maintenance needs.

A top-ranked EHR should be integrated – not interfaced – with a first-rate practice management system, because revenue cycle management is the lifeblood of any physician practice. And as patients assume greater financial responsibility for their care, new point of care patient payment tools will be required to facilitate collection. One such tool enables practices to calculate how much a patient is likely to owe after insurance coverage and obtain payment by credit or debit card before the patient leaves the office. The most advanced EHR/PM systems are also integrated with software that enables patients to pay their bills online, reducing the percentage of self-pay accounts that must be written off as bad debt.

Finally, to help practices ramp up to obtain full government incentives by the 2011 deadline, EHR providers must find ways to accelerate implementation. One approach that can be helpful is to use physician designed "certified workflows" that require less customization, along with configuration "wizards" that enable practices to set their own parameters with less outside help than is now typically the case. Advanced distance learning modules can supplement onsite training and enable busy physicians to learn how to use the EHR at their own pace. Taken together, these innovations can significantly reduce the total number of "effort hours" needed to implement our EHR.

The Future of EHRs

Interoperability among EHRs and other information systems will develop rapidly as a result of both the meaningful use rules and the federal funding of state and regional health information exchanges (HIEs). When most providers can exchange data online across all care settings, that capability will revolutionize health care and lead us toward dramatically higher quality and lower costs, just as the Internet connected computers, and changed the way we do everything.

Physicians would do well to remember that the goal is not "one system" but rather "one patient record."

To take connectivity to a higher level, EHRs of the future will need to have universal connectivity across the spectrum of care. Electronic prescribing is already close to that point, because Surescripts has made it possible for most pharmacies to accept online prescriptions over its network. Lab connectivity is a bigger challenge for practices.

EHRs of the future will also be expected to include features that help physicians compete for pay-for-performance, pay-for-quality, and pay-for-value bonuses that will become a major part of their reimbursement. These will include not only registry functions but also more sophisticated decision support that will help physicians fine-tune treatment plans for particular patients, derived from the latest evidence-based medicine and, in the near future, the patient's genome.

The user interfaces of EHRs will also continue to evolve, making it easier for physicians to work with computers. To reduce the time investment associated with data entry – long an obstacle to EHR adoption – alternative methods of entering discrete data into our EHRs will be needed including voice, handwriting recognition, and self service from patients entering their own information.

In the end, the goal of EHR adoption is to improve the health of patients and the financial "health" of our healthcare system. Our vision is to provide a connected system of health by supplying our physicians with the best information when and where they need it, and connecting them with all of the other healthcare stakeholders in their communities. Together, information and connectivity enable physicians to deliver better care while making their work day easier and more satisfying. Thanks to the strong partnerships we have developed with our clients, it is a vision that is being realized today in multiple communities across the country.

Ambulatory Electronic Medical Records for Today and Tomorrow – A Cerner Physician's Perspective

DR. ROBERT BART Chief Medical Officer and Director, Client Corporation

DR. ROBERT BART is chief medical officer and director responsible for client development in the children's and academic segments of Cerner Corporation. He joined Cerner in 2007, bringing with him 15 years of pediatric critical care medicine experience and 5 years of clinical information technology experience.

Physicians purchasing an ambulatory EHR system to automate their practice are doing so at a very exciting time. In early 2009, the federal government passed the American Recovery and Reinvestment Act (ARRA), ushering in an era of unprecedented government support for moving healthcare delivery to an electronic platform. Those who are purchasing an EHR today not only need to consider physician workflow and productivity, but also to be mindful of the Centers for Medicare and Medicaid Services (CMS) definition of "meaningful use." Although meaningful use is an evolving standard, once defined, it will be the minimum data set and functionality the government expects from an EHR. The definition of meaningful use will be meted out in three phases beginning in 2011. Through these evolving standards, the federal government has provided the present-day "carrot" and future "stick" for moving healthcare from paper-based to digital documentation. With the passage of this legislation, it is essential that hospitals, multi-specialty groups, and solo practitioners convert to EHRs.

Prior to ARRA, physicians considering an EHR for their practice only had to concern themselves with a simple test drive and evaluation prior to purchasing. Today, these same physicians also need to consider usability as well as sustainability over time and the ability of the EHR to meet CMS regulations. Physicians must look for a solution supplier that

1. has the ability to keep up with evolving regulatory reporting requirements;
2. offers an application service provider (ASP) model that frees the provider to focus on clinical care, taking the burden of technology management off the physician's shoulders;
3. allow for management at both a single-patient and population level; and
4. integrate and interoperate with other solutions.

Physicians will also have two macro concerns as adoption of technology within the healthcare industry advances. First, physicians must partner with a supplier that is focused on innovation. Areas of focus should include supporting the evolution of the ambulatory physician workflow, usability, optimizing patient care, and physician efficiency. Information technology from these suppliers also should be able to facilitate the communication and engagement of the patient outside the traditional clinical care settings, and it should provide enhanced continuity and care coordination across the spectrum of healthcare venues.

Secondly, physicians must identify an information technology supplier that has a proven track record of collaborating with its clients. It is beneficial if the supplier is a publicly traded corporation that is open to giving physicians insights into its business model and the monetary amount it invests in research and development.

As mentioned, meaningful use is an overriding focus for physicians purchasing an EHR system today. Although meaningful use requirements are still under development at the writing of this piece, it is clear that the definition more clearly favors the functional certification approach taken by Certification Commission for Health Information Technology (CCHIT) over the Healthcare Information and Management Systems Society (HIMSS) analytics model of EHR adoption. There are some high-level tenets of functionality that can be gleaned from early versions of meaningful use and previous functional certifications performed by CCHIT: patient access to their medical information, maintenance of privacy and security, the ability to share information electronically to patient-authorized providers, foundational elements of clinical outcome reporting, real-time clinical decision support, and the inclusion of patient preferences in prescribing practices. In addition, industry watchdog KLAS authored a report, "Meaningful use leading to improved outcomes," which should be required reading prior to purchasing an EHR.

In the future, practicing physicians will see an ever-increasing dependency on EHR systems for all aspects of their medical practice. The EHR will become the physician's HIPPA-compliant communication hub. It will be able to securely exchange medical information with all aspects of the healthcare industry, including the consumer. In this vein, EHR suppliers should be able to move medical information in an interoperable manner through technology-agnostic information exchanges – through a healthcare hub if you will. Additionally, the physician's EHR should be able to report test results to the patient's personal health record and to provide information, daily guidance, and goals in a personalized manner.

Moving beyond the clinical functionality of the EHR, additional decision points fall to the physician's personal considerations and circumstance. Even within an ASP model of EHR delivery, the physician needs to understand how the solution supplier handles technical support and problem resolution. Depending on the ambulatory physician's practice setting and given the loosening of Stark restrictions, a neighboring hospital may help pay for the physicians EHR. The physician should also ask if the IT system can support business office and practice management needs. The physician should account for practice growth – both of providers currently using an EHR and of providers who may join the practice in the future. In short, a physician or provider group needs a nimble EHR system that can flex with their size and needs as the practice or the future of medicine changes.

Earlier, I stated that CMS will issue the definition of meaningful use in three phases – in 2011, 2013, and 2015. It is these future requirements and the government's "stick" in the form of decrementing healthcare service reimbursements to the provider that will drive ongoing adherence to meaningful use. Broadly, I believe these future requirements not only will contain directives for additional functionality within the EHR, but also will push EHR systems into becoming part of a larger interoperable integrated healthcare network. Currently, such a network enhances communications between the consumer/patient, ambulatory healthcare providers, hospitals, pharmacies, and other healthcare entities. In the future, this network will expand to include information gathering and learning. Such a healthcare learning network will be able to identify community, county, state, regional and national disease, and condition trends. This network will enable rapid evidence generation and knowledge dissemination, and it will integrate laboratory tests, clinical documentation, and medication ordering practices. Coinciding with this healthcare learning network, there will be changes in reporting processes to CMS and other healthcare regulatory and quality agencies. Reporting will change from a manual push process to an automated pull from the EHR, taking the burden of manual reporting off of clinicians. Analysis of this information will add to our understanding of disease and condition epidemiology. Importantly, physician reimbursements will become more directly linked to outcomes and the quality of care provided. This linkage should improve healthcare for the consumer and become part of a more economical healthcare model.

Healthcare also will see a transition from population-derived interventions and therapies to personalized medicine – with personalized interventions, therapies, and treatment plans. Eventually, we will unveil how a lifetime of environmental exposure, personal intent, and desires affect each individual's genome. In advance of this information, the EHR needs to have a data structure that allows for the insertion and storage of patient-specific information. This placeholder technology enables today's EHR to grow as the information collected on each patient changes and grows in complexity.

Ultimately, a knowledgeable and thoughtful EHR selection should only happen once during the lifetime of a practitioner or a clinical practice. The physician or practice should start with the identification of publicly traded corporations that maintain financial transparency with their clients and offer an ASP model ambulatory EHR solution. Add to these criteria the requirements provided by CMS on meaningful use, physician usability, practice management, integrated interoperability, genomic data capture, and environmental history you should have the guidance you need for selecting an EHR for today's world and tomorrow's.

Practice Considerations for Purchasing EHR

EHR Must Help – Not Complicate – The Lives of the Solo or Small-Group Practitioners

Robert Quinn, *Executive Vice President, Chief Technology Officer, Epocrates*

Robert Quinn has 20 years of experience as an engineer and software development manager. Prior to joining Epocrates, Bob served as VP of Engineering for iDini Corporation, a wireless software startup, and was instrumental in the growth and acquisition of Inpart Design, an internet-based engineering services company that is now part of PTC. Previously, Bob held a variety of technical and engineering-management positions with IBM. He received his bachelor's from Dartmouth College, holds a Ph.D. from the University of Colorado, and was a research fellow at Harvard University prior to joining IBM.

Long before the US government offered financial incentives to incorporate EHRs into medical practices, many physicians were using digital technologies in their professional lives to help manage the escalating demands on their practices. Under pressure from higher patient volume and lower reimbursement rates, doctors turned to both the Web and mobile devices to improve efficiencies, particularly in how they accessed drug information and decision support tools, and how they communicated with partners, vendors, and patients. The EHR represents the next step in the natural progression toward the advancement of healthcare. In fact, broader adoption of EHR will be instrumental in helping physicians respond to continued demand for reductions in healthcare costs, fewer medical errors, and improvements in measurable outcomes.

The trend toward greater use of digital tools has set the stage for a dramatic increase in EHR adoption. The willingness of medical professionals to turn to newer digital technologies is underscored by the following numbers:

- The average doctor spent twice as many hours online in 2009 compared to 2003
- 75% of physicians go online daily
- One-third of medical professionals use the Web during patient consults
- 90% of MDs report that the Internet is essential to their practice
- Two-thirds have mobile devices; 70% of users state that their smart phone or PDA is likewise essential

Source: *Physicians in 2012,* Manhattan Research, LLC, ©2009, 2010

The recent Medicare incentive to reward physicians who demonstrate "meaningful use" of EHR provides yet another stimulus for rapid conversion to these cutting-edge systems. Of course, "meaningful use" will need to be more precisely defined. Significant progress has already been made in the subsequent debate among stakeholders. The Office of the National Coordinator for Health Information Technology (ONCHIT) is expected to issue final policies and standards sometime in 2010. These eagerly awaited guidelines will further fuel adoption.

EHR: The Haves and the Have-Nots

EHR has already secured a significant foothold within the medical community. According to the 2010 Manhattan Research report, *Physicians in 2012 (Part 2): The Outlook on Health Information Technology*, approximately 40% of physicians – largely in hospital settings – currently use an EHR and 10% are in the process of implementing a system. However, fully half of medical practices are not yet engaged in adopting a technology that is redefining health-care delivery.

To fully realize the efficiencies and improved outcomes made possible by EHR, the US healthcare system must secure the participation of a broader spectrum of medical practices. EHR early adopters are predominantly institutions and large- or medium-sized medical offices. Uptake by small and solo practices is low. For example, only 11% of current users are doctors in solo practices. Of physicians with no plans to incorporate EHR, nearly half are solo practitioners.

Numerous obstacles dissuade solo and small-practice physicians from joining the EHR revolution, including

- **Cost:** Despite government incentives, the cost of EHR can still be prohibitive. In addition to the initial purchase, start-up and maintenance may add further expense. For this reason, physicians must carefully select a system that provides real value to their practices.
- **Practice disruption:** Busy physicians and their overworked small staffs have little time to learn and integrate new systems. Likewise, they have few resources for in-house training. Although EHR can offer significant long-term efficiencies to operations of any size, the wrong system can have an immediate negative effect on workflow.
- **Confusion over best vendor:** How does a small or solo practice decide which EHR vendor best meets its needs? Every practice functions somewhat differently has its own individualized mix of strengths and shortcomings and may require varying degrees of support for its EHR function. Unlike a comprehensive practice that can field its own tech-support team, the smaller operation will need a reliable EHR partner that delivers a versatile yet convenient system that meets its functional needs in a highly usable fashion.

Fortunately, there are many options from which to choose. Unfortunately, the sheer number of systems can make it difficult for the average small practice to evaluate and select the optimal one. What is a doctor to do?

EHR Selection Criteria

The following will help ensure that small and solo practices make wise EHR purchases:

- **Utility:** What features of EHR matter to you most? Physicians are in the business of patient care. A key value of an EHR is to help you improve patient care by flagging drug interactions, safety issues, and information exchange within the continuum of care. If you are in a small practice, look for an EHR that is geared to meet the needs of a small practice. Look for an EHR that allows users to migrate at its own pace, providing the option to print records and file in existing charts.
- **Versatility:** Every practice is unique and an EHR system should be as adaptable as your practice. It should also be well-designed with interfaces that are tuned for both desktop and mobile platforms. To ensure its EHR system responds to the issues that matter most small practitioners, look for an EHR where the developers are using a physician-driven – instead of engineer-driven – process where doctors with particular expertise in health-information technology are core members of the development team. At each design phase, software should be beta-tested extensively by doctors out in the field, and their feedback incorporated to guarantee that the system addresses real-life practice demands.

- **Integration:** If your practice is limited in size, odds are that you do not have an IT staff that can oversee complex installation. Therefore, your EHR should be compatible with your existing platforms and as close to plug-and-play as possible. It should also have a familiar interface based on software conventions so that it is easily accessible to any professional with basic computer skills. Who has time for extensive training or technical support calls when they are focused on caring for patients? Convenient online resources should be available to get users up to speed quickly and walk them through simple solutions or common concerns.
- **Reputation:** Is your EHR vendor a newcomer riding the wave of the next hot business opportunity, or a committed partner with a long-history and proven track record for quality products and service? EHR solutions should clearly be based on a fundamental understanding of the growing digital-communications needs of today's medical practices.

EHR technology is instrumental to fulfilling the primary objectives of today's rapidly evolving healthcare delivery system, including practice efficiency, error reduction, cost savings, care coordination and, ultimately, improved patient outcomes. To achieve these benefits, EHR systems must be practical and accessible to physicians in offices of all sizes. The specific challenges facing small and solo practices can often be overwhelming, yet their successful integration into the "digitized" medical system is critical. EHR technology must help – not complicate – its contribution.

Subject Index

N.S. Skolnik (ed.), *Electronic Medical Records*, Current Clinical Practice,
DOI 10.1007/978-1-60761-606-1, © Springer Science+Business Media, LLC 2011

Made in the USA
San Bernardino, CA
02 March 2018